THE
CBD
BOOK

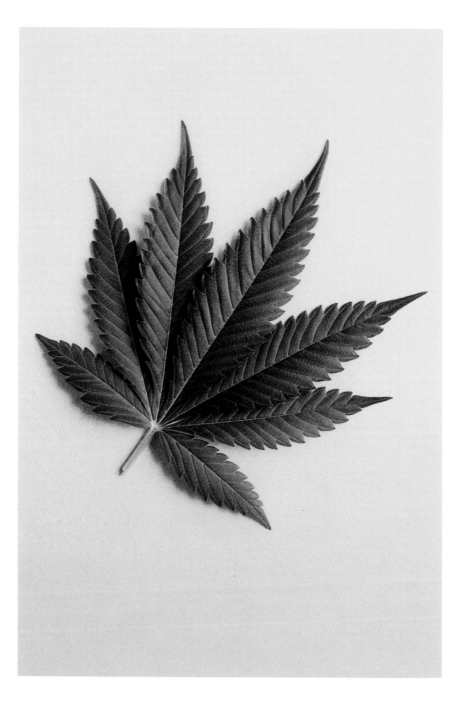

MARY BILES

THE
ESSENTIAL
GUIDE TO
CBD OIL

THE
CBD
BOOK

Thorsons

CONTENTS

04. CBD FOR WELLNESS

05. HOW TO TAKE CBD

06. CASE STUDIES

IN MEMORY OF CHARLOTTE FIGI

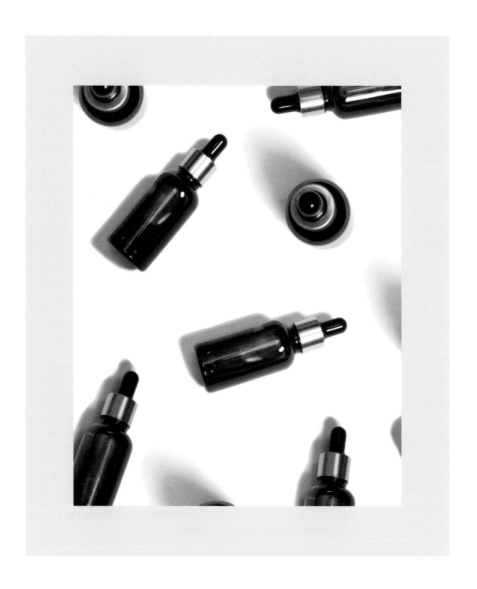

FOREWORD

It was the early 2000s; I had recently been awarded my PhD, and had been given funds to start up a new research group. I was keen for the research to be translational, so I approached a number of clinicians to identify areas where science could supplement clinical observations. One doctor came up to me and mentioned how an increasing number of his patients were smoking cannabis while on their chemotherapy. This innocuous remark led to a research journey into the activities of the active ingredients in the cannabis plant, which has helped us to understand the complex nature of these compounds.

There is no doubt that a number of these compounds possess biological activity – the number of phone calls that I get every day from patients using them attests to that. It does not take long for people to read how phytocannabinoids such as CBD have helped with their diseases. They feel this is their way to tackle their own disease. However, a common theme of these calls is the lack of good, concise information. Answers to fundamental questions are desperately needed.

This book provides answers to these questions about CBD: what is it, how does it work and more importantly, is it right for me? It has been written by Mary, whom I have known for about a year. She has interviewed me a number of times about

my work, and I have been impressed by the style of her writing. She has the journalistic flair to deconvolute a subject; to identify the key parts of the narrative, and then to present it in a way that is easy to grasp. It is not enough to just have a knack for documenting a story, you need to immerse yourself in it; Mary has explored this field for a number of years, which has given her an insight to what people really want and need to know.

Dr Wai Liu
Senior Research Fellow
St George's, University of London

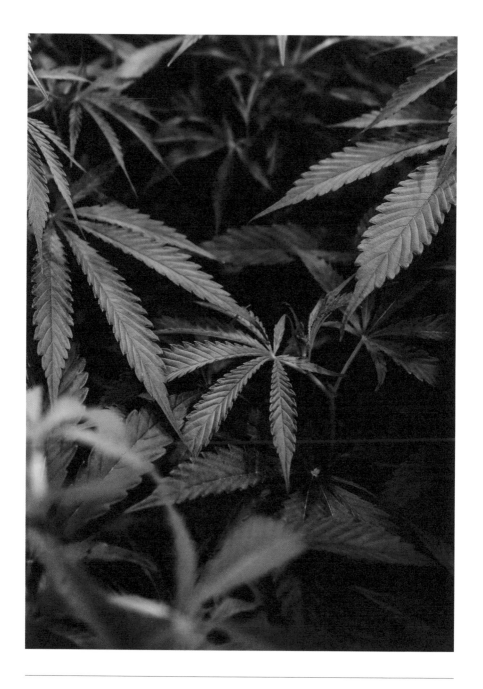

THE CBD BOOK

INTRODUCTION

If you're reading this book, it's almost certainly because you're 'CBD-curious' or already taking CBD products. Perhaps you've googled 'buy CBD' and found yourself bamboozled by the dizzying array of CBD companies all claiming to have the best-quality CBD oil on the market.

Then there's the question of which type of CBD product to buy. Should you go the CBD oil route, choose CBD capsules, CBD topicals or even vape it? And it's not like CBD is easy on the pocket, so making the right choice and not coming away with some kind of snake oil is incredibly important.

I am not a doctor and I won't be giving any medical advice in this book. However, as the resident CBD expert on the block, I can't tell you how many times I get asked for tips on how to navigate the complicated maze of CBD companies and their products.

Next comes the clear-as-mud instructions on how much CBD to take. With medication and health supplements, we're used to getting precise dosing instructions; being told to start low and go slow while listening to our body is something we are just not accustomed to.

But this is just the invitation I make to anyone embarking on their CBD adventure. It is an opportunity to get better acquainted with ourselves, asking what our bodies and minds really need right now. For many, CBD can be a real game changer, facilitating a feeling of wellbeing not experienced for a long time. That said, CBD is not a panacea and for others it may not have such an effect.

However, it's imperative to start from a baseline of choosing a product that is clean, safe, free from any hidden nasties such as pesticides, heavy metals and mould, and more importantly, contains precisely the amount of CBD it says on the label.

This may sound obvious, but in 2019 the Centre for Medical Cannabis tested 30 CBD products found on the high street and online. Only 38 per cent contained within 10 per cent of the CBD advertised and one high-street pharmacy CBD oil had no CBD at all. Another CBD product contained 3.8 per cent alcohol, qualifying it as an alcoholic beverage.[1] Shocking, right?

At present, the CBD market is at best self-regulated, and at worst a kind of hemp Wild West. As a consumer, it is almost impossible to know the reputable, compliant companies from the dodgier variants on the market.

This is where I, as author of *The CBD Book*, come in. After a varied career spent in TV production, journalism and complementary therapies, fate brought me in contact with the medicinal properties of cannabis and hemp. Before I knew it, I was immersed in the CBD industry, interviewing top cannabinoid scientists and writing for one of the original European CBD pioneers. It was very much a baptism of fire, but I came out the other end with an insider's knowledge that I want to share with you, the CBD consumer.

Reading *The CBD Book* will give you invaluable tips from an industry expert to help guide you through the confusing process of incorporating CBD oil into your day-to-day life – whether it's for wellness reasons or because you hope CBD may help with the more complex needs associated with illness.

HOW TO USE THIS BOOK

To get the most benefits from both the book and CBD oil itself, it's important to understand how CBD interacts with the body, as well as having a realistic view of current scientific research. Therefore, I recommend reading the book in order, although it's also OK to cherry-pick the chapters that most resonate with you and your needs.

If science isn't your thing, don't panic. As a writer (and non-scientist), my modus operandi is to be a bridge between the big-brained molecular biology types and ordinary people like you and me who just want to understand how CBD might be beneficial to our health.

So, I do recommend spending some time reading the 'CBD Basics' chapter (see pages 21–32), in particular the sections on the endocannabinoid system, which I will return to at various points in the book, especially when I cover CBD research.

'How To Take CBD' (see pages 83–114) is an important section for getting a practical handle on how to choose the best CBD product for you, and it will clear up any confusion about the different types of CBD products on the market. Questions about how to find the right dosage and potential drug interactions will also be covered.

Finally, to get a true sense of how CBD can empower people's lives, I strongly recommend reading the series of case studies (see pages 115–126).

Whichever way you choose to enjoy the book, incorporating CBD into your life will take you on an exciting journey of self-discovery. A journey I am delighted to join you on.

'Reading *The CBD Book* will give you invaluable tips from an industry expert to help guide you through the confusing process of incorporating CBD oil into your life.'

01

THE HISTORY OF CBD

From Zero to Hero

If you'd told me five years ago I'd be educating the world about a compound in cannabis called CBD, I'd have said you're out of your mind. That's because back then CBD, or cannabidiol as it's officially known, was barely heard of outside medical cannabis communities in Colorado and California. These days, CBD oil can be found on most high streets, where health-food stores, pharmacies and even supermarkets are stocking CBD products. And we're not just talking your bog-standard CBD oil drops. Oh no, CBD can be found in everything from cocktails, coffee, beer, hummus, bath bombs, mascara, moisturiser and even ladies' active wear.

CBD is literally everywhere and everyone wants to get in on the act. This shouldn't be a huge surprise when you consider the global CBD market is predicted to be worth $16 billion by 2025.[2]

Current estimates suggest 8 to 11 per cent of Brits[3] and 14 per cent of Americans[4] have tried CBD oil, and this number looks set to rise even further.

Perhaps CBD's most vocal fans have been the host of A-list celebrities singing its praises. Kim Kardashian threw a CBD-themed baby shower; Jennifer Aniston uses CBD to help with stress and anxiety; and Mandy Moore protected her feet against an unforgiving red carpet by rubbing CBD oil into her heels.

But how did CBD go from a cannabis nobody to a global wellness phenomenon?

A POTTED HISTORY OF CBD

AND MEDICAL CANNABIS

CBD as a compound was only discovered 80 years ago. However, it has been present in the cannabis used medicinally and in our diet throughout history. That's why in order to tell the CBD story, we must consider the historical use of cannabis as a whole.

Cannabis and hemp have been used as a medicine, a source of food and a durable fibre for thousands of years. In 2900 BC, Chinese Emperor Fu Hsi was first to mention the medicinal properties of cannabis, but since then it has been pretty much part of the pharmacopoeias of all civilisations, including the Egyptians, the Ancient Greeks and the Romans.

In the 19th century, using cannabis medicinally became widespread after the Irish physician William O'Shaughnessy returned to European shores with knowledge gained from his time in India. Rumour has it, Queen Victoria was even given cannabis by her doctor to treat menstrual cramps.

CANNABIS DISAPPEARS FROM OUR MEDICINE CABINET

At the beginning of the 20th century, it wouldn't have been unusual for doctors to prescribe cannabis tinctures for everything from headaches to rheumatic pains or convulsions. However, just a decade later in post-prohibition America, the newly appointed head of the Federal Bureau of Narcotics, Harry Anslinger, turned his attention to demonising cannabis. And so began a relentless campaign linking cannabis to all societal ills, fuelled by Anslinger's own prejudice against people of colour and Mexicans, who were the predominant cannabis users at the time.

With the passing of the Anslinger-drafted 1937 Marihuana Tax Act, it became effectively illegal to sell cannabis medicinal products in pharmacies in the United States, and with this began 70 years of cannabis prohibition.[5]

The US was not alone in its bid to wipe the world clean of cannabis. In 1961, 185 countries signed the Single Convention on Narcotic drugs, committing themselves to limiting the consumption, possession and trafficking of narcotic drugs to medical and scientific purposes. With pressure from the United States, the convention included cannabis in both Schedule 1 and Schedule 4; a classification reserved for drugs such as heroin that pose serious risk of abuse and have limited therapeutic value.[6]

Member states like the USA and UK subsequently fulfilled their treaty obligations, introducing the 1970 Controlled Substance Act[7] and 1971 Misuse of Drugs Act[8] respectively, classifying cannabis as dangerous and without medicinal benefit.

What does this have to do with CBD, you may ask? Well, CBD is a compound found in *Cannabis sativa* – the Latin term for what we know as cannabis, marijuana and hemp. We now know that CBD does not get us high, but Anslinger and his cronies neither understood nor cared about the complexities of the cannabis plant; they were just intent on banning it outright.

Sadly, a consequence of this 70-year global cannabis prohibition has been the stifling of crucial research into all the plant's constituent parts, including CBD, as well as an overall stigmatisation of cannabis as medicine.

THE DISCOVERY OF CBD

The scientific world has known about CBD since 1940, when American organic chemist Roger Adams discovered CBD (cannabidiol) in his lab. In 1963, Professor Raphael Mechoulam, affectionately known as the grandfather of cannabis science, mapped out CBD's structure, and in 1965 became the first scientist to synthesise CBD.[9]

It was Mechoulam who initially shone a light on CBD's medicinal potential. In 1980, he gave the compound to eight patients with epilepsy over four and a half months.[10] Four subjects were almost seizure free during the study and three others noted significant improvement. Plus, CBD was found to be non-toxic and free from serious side effects. Professor Mechoulam was convinced this would be the beginning of a CBD revolution in medicine, but it took another 25 years for these studies to be taken seriously.

That's not to say CBD's brain-protecting potential had gone unnoticed. In 2003, the US government was granted a patent for the use of CBD as a neuroprotectant and antioxidant in neurodegenerative diseases and strokes.[11] A somewhat perplexing position when you consider that federally cannabis was considered without any accepted medical benefit.

But what was laid down by federal law was not necessarily followed by certain states within the US, and in 1996 California became the first state to legalise medical cannabis, followed two years later by Colorado and Oregon.

'A consequence of this global cannabis prohibition has been the stifling of crucial research.'

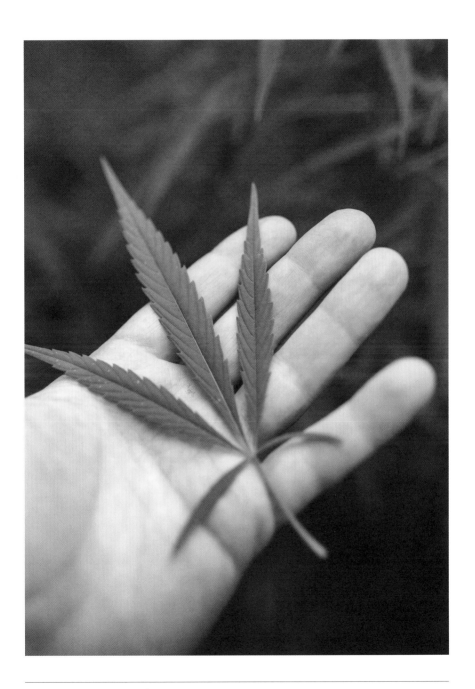

CHILD WITH EPILEPSY INTRODUCES CBD TO THE WORLD

While CBD made it into California's medical marijuana programme in 2009, in the annals of CBD history, Colorado could be considered the birthplace of its current boom. Around the same time the Stanley Brothers, five clean-living Christian brothers, tentatively entered the world of medical marijuana after they began giving cannabis oil to patients with cancer and multiple sclerosis in Colorado.

They went on to open a couple of dispensaries, but had trouble shifting one particular cannabis oil they'd christened 'hippies' disappointment'. High levels of CBD and virtually no THC meant the cannabis oil had no intoxicating effect, and was of little interest to the majority of customers.

However, it proved to be a game changer for Colorado resident Paige Figi, mother of five-year-old Charlotte, who had been researching the anticonvulsant effects of CBD. Little Charlotte had a rare epileptic condition called Dravet Syndrome, which saw her suffering upwards of 300 seizures a week. Unresponsive to conventional treatment, Charlotte's cognitive development had been severely impaired and it was likely a huge seizure could end her life at any time.

In desperation, Paige turned to the Stanley Brothers who gave her their CBD oil to try. In what seemed like a miracle, Charlotte's seizures dramatically reduced, and soon the word got out to the parents of other children with epilepsy.

However, it was in 2013 when CNN's health correspondent Dr Sanjay Gupta made the documentary 'Weeds' featuring Charlotte's story, that CBD oil went truly mainstream.

EUROPE TURNS HEMP INTO A CBD GOLDMINE

Like anything cannabis-related, the UK and Europe took a while to catch up with the CBD oil trend sweeping the US.

By 2014, a few European early pioneers were selling CBD oils. Made from industrial hemp, these CBD products contained only trace amounts of THC, the illegal part of cannabis responsible for the high. Hemp had been grown for its durable fibre and nutritious seeds in Europe for hundreds of years; however, using hemp flowers to make CBD oil was a new departure.

As knowledge emerged about the health-giving properties of CBD, a few savvy individuals realised this could be an innovative way to make cannabis oil legally available to the general public. And with that, the European CBD industry was born.

In the UK, the Home Office does not permit farmers to cultivate hemp flowers and buds, which remain 'controlled' parts of the plant. Unfortunately, only small amounts of CBD are found in hemp leaves and stalks, so most CBD oil companies source their products from European-grown hemp.

CBD GETS REGULATED (SORT OF)

Back then, CBD oil was talked about in hushed tones and was almost exclusively sold on the internet. Companies waxed lyrical about CBD's seemingly miraculous powers to heal almost any ailment, including the scary ones like cancer. This caught the attention of the UK's Medicines and Healthcare Products Regulatory Agency (MHRA), an executive agency of the Department of Health and Social Care responsible for ensuring that medicines are effective and safe.

Medical claims can only be made for products licensed (usually pharmaceutical drugs) by the MHRA, the European Medicines Agency (EMA) or the United States Food and Drug Administration (FDA). Authorisation is a lengthy and costly process involving three stages of clinical trials. CBD oils sold on the market as food supplements back then have not been through any of these processes.

However, Sativex, a cannabis-based pharmaceutical drug containing CBD (and THC) was already approved by the MHRA for multiple sclerosis patients. The MHRA were also aware of a growing body of scientific research suggesting CBD may treat certain diseases and could therefore be considered a medicine.

So, in October 2016, the MHRA concluded that 'products containing cannabidiol (CBD) used for medical purposes are a medicine'.

This meant that CBD companies had to immediately remove any medical claims from their marketing materials in order to continue selling their products. This is the reason why reputable CBD companies will never suggest CBD cures or treats health conditions on their websites or packaging.

Similar warnings have been issued by the FDA in the United States. However, the situation there is rather more complicated. As a compound extracted from cannabis, CBD continues to be classified as a Schedule 1 drug by the US Federal Government and, as such, is not approved as a prescription drug or dietary supplement and is not allowed to be sold interstate. However, in states where some form of medical cannabis has been legalised, CBD oil is as ubiquitous – if not more so – than the UK.

One of the chief concerns of agencies like the FDA and the Food Standards Agency (FSA) in the UK, is whether CBD oil products are safe to be consumed by the public. In several countries, including the US and the UK, a cross section of CBD oils have been tested and in general the amount of CBD oil advertised on the label is not reflected in the product. In many cases, more than the legal limit of THC (0.3 per cent in the US and 0.2 per cent in the UK) can be found, which, as well as potentially causing unwanted intoxication, could lead to consumers failing drug tests.

CHANGING ATTITUDES
TO CBD

The World Health Organisation (WHO) reported their own findings on CBD in their 2018 Critical Review Report.[12] They found CBD to be well tolerated with a good safety profile, free from any risk of addiction or abuse, and acknowledged its clinical use in childhood epilepsy. However, the report mostly referred to purified CBD used in scientific research rather than CBD-based products sold to consumers.

In 2018, there were also some big changes on either side of the Atlantic. In the UK, CBD went on sale in the high-street health-food store Holland and Barrett, instantly becoming one of their most popular products. Pharmacies and supermarkets followed suit, making CBD accessible to consumers who felt uncomfortable buying their CBD oil online.

In the United States, the 2018 Farm Bill successfully removed hemp (*Cannabis sativa* containing less than 0.3 per cent THC) from the list of Schedule 1 controlled substances. Finally, hemp was just another agricultural commodity that could be grown legally by farmers and transported across state lines. In the past, hemp could only be cultivated with special licences for scientific research, so most of the CBD oil available in the US came from European-grown hemp. Following the Farm Bill, companies can now make their CBD oils from 100 per cent American-grown hemp.

Does this mean CBD is now legal state-wide? Well, not exactly. At a federal level, CBD continues to be a Schedule 1 controlled substance and hemp-derived CBD is only legal if the hemp is produced in a manner consistent not only with the Farm Bill but also associated federal and state regulations, and is produced by a licensed grower.

There was also a historic moment in the UK in 2018, when the government agreed to reclassify cannabis-based medicinal products to Schedule 2, making it possible for doctors to prescribe cannabis to patients. However, this does not have any direct impact on the CBD nutritional supplement market, as these products cannot be prescribed by physicians.

FIRST CBD PHARMACEUTICAL DRUG APPROVED

Almost 40 years after Raphael Mechoulam's pioneering study using CBD to reduce seizures in patients with epilepsy, the British biopharmaceutical company GW Pharma finally got authorisation to market its antiseizure drug, Epidyolex. Containing purified CBD, Epidyolex had successfully passed through the lengthy and expensive randomised clinical trials for two rare classes of drug-resistant epilepsy: Dravet and Lennox-Gastaut syndromes.

Epidyolex thus became the first cannabis-based drug to be approved in the United States and is also available in Europe. However, in the UK, NICE has restricted Epidyolex to Dravet and Lennox-Gastaut Syndromes.

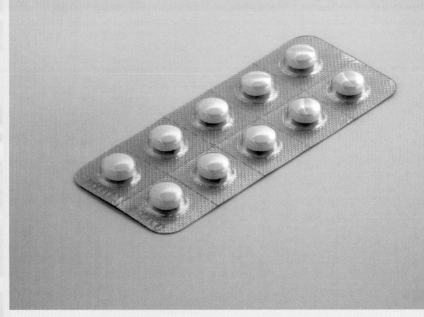

IS CBD TOO NOVEL FOR FOODS?

The ever-shifting sands of the CBD industry saw the European Food Safety Authority (EFSA) throw a particular curveball when it included CBD (and other cannabinoids) in their catalogue of novel foods in 2019.[13]

A food is classed as novel if it wasn't regularly consumed before 1997. Despite protestations from the CBD industry about CBD's consumption in hemp over hundreds if not thousands of years, its entry in the novel food catalogue means authorisations are required to prove CBD's safety for human consumption in food and nutritional supplements.

The UK's Food Standards Agency (FSA) has stated their position, warning they will crack down on CBD companies who haven't submitted valid novel food applications by 31 March 2021. What this means in effect is that any non-compliant CBD products will be removed from shelves by trading standards officers and there will be a natural slimming down of the CBD industry.

In the United States, because CBD is the subject of an Investigational New Drug Application (for Epidiolex) and was not previously marketed in foods, it cannot be legally added to comestibles (including nutritional supplements).

So far, only the states of Washington, North Carolina, Ohio and the city of New York have banned businesses from selling food and drink containing CBD. However, with a plethora of CBD oils, edibles and drinks on the market elsewhere, it would seem most CBD companies are choosing to ignore FDA regulations.

It can sometimes feel like forces greater than ourselves are conspiring to limit CBD's global expansion as both a wellness product and as medicine. Most agree that more regulation is necessary to weed out the less reputable CBD operators. However, this could mean only the big players who can afford the expensive licenses and authorisations required to sell CBD will remain.

Either way, it can be guaranteed that the next five years will see an equally dizzying amount of change in the CBD market. So hold onto your hats, it's going to be an exciting ride!

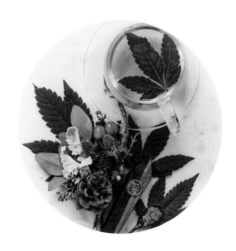

02

CBD
BASICS

Snake Oil or Miracle Cure?

Depending on whom you speak to, CBD is described as anything from a snake oil to a miracle cure and everything in between.

It's true that in some cases the same CBD oil products reducing seizures in children with epilepsy are also popular in the wellness sector, something unheard of in the nutritional supplement market until now. That's why CBD is increasingly known as a health industry disruptor.

It may also explain why many fear that the pharmaceutical industry is looking for ways to close the CBD oil sector down. After all, if instead of swallowing a handful of prescription meds, patients are popping to the health food store to buy a side-effect-free and often more effective natural alternative, this will not go down well in big pharma board meetings.

That said, CBD oil is not a panacea. Some people find that they feel their health has improved after taking it, while others notice no difference at all. In the end, CBD is like any other wellness product or even pharmaceutical drug: it will work for some people and not for others.

But if we're to really get a handle on how best to harness CBD's therapeutic potential, it's vital to get to grips with some CBD fundamentals. So, welcome to our CBD basics.

WHAT IS CBD?

Head to any website about CBD and it can feel like you're bombarded with a load of scientific terms that you would need a degree in molecular biology to make any sense of.

What's the point of all that fancy-pants science stuff if all you want to do is take some CBD and feel less stressed? I might have said the same thing a few years ago, but it's actually quite fun getting a rudimentary understanding of CBD and how it affects the body.

CBD, otherwise known as cannabidiol, is one of 144 cannabinoids[14], which are a special class of compounds predominantly found and produced in the sticky trichomes of cannabis flowers.

While tetrahydrocannabinol (THC), the bit that gets you stoned, has traditionally been the most abundant cannabinoid in cannabis, depending on the cannabis strain, varying amounts of CBD can also be found.

Hemp, which is still cannabis, just with only trace levels of THC, tends to have more CBD. That's why in countries where THC is illegal (in effect, most of the world), CBD is extracted from hemp plants (sometimes called industrial hemp).

Other types of cannabinoids include: tetrahydrocannabinolic acid (THCA), cannabinol (CBN), cannabigerol (CBG), cannabichromene (CBC), tetrahydrocannabivarin (THCV), and cannabidiolic acid (CBDA), all of which interact with the body in different ways.

CBDA is particularly interesting because it is CBD's acidic precursor. Contrary to what you might imagine, unpicked hemp contains very little CBD, but it is abundant in CBDA. When CBDA is dried or heated it is converted into CBD through a process known as decarboxylation (the removal of a carboxyl group). CBDA is an interesting cannabinoid in its own right, showing potential as an anticonvulsant and anti-nausea drug, and many CBD oils contain both CBD and CBDA.

A challenging aspect of CBD is the fact that it is lipophilic, meaning it tends to combine with or dissolve in fats rather than water. Seeing as our bodies contain 60 per cent water, much of the CBD taken orally cannot be absorbed by our bodies. Consequently, a lot of research and development is happening right now, looking into more efficient ways of ingesting CBD. But more on that later.

CBD IS SAFE

The good news is that scientific research has shown that even at high doses (up to 2000mg per day in some cases), CBD doesn't have any serious side effects.[15] Most people take between 10–50mg of CBD a day (assuming their CBD oil contains the amount of CBD it says on the label). So it's unlikely the side effects (drowsiness, reduced appetite, diarrhoea, and fatigue) experienced by the children with epilepsy who were given up to 50mg per kilo of body weight of pure CBD, will be repeated at lower doses.

CBD WILL NOT MAKE YOU FEEL STONED

For many people taking CBD oil, this is the first direct experience they've ever had with cannabis. 'Will I feel stoned?' and 'can I become addicted?' are questions that are often asked.

The good news is that CBD is not going to make you feel high, stoned or any of those altered states associated with recreational cannabis. However, this doesn't mean that CBD is classed as non-psychoactive.

Psychoactive is defined as a substance (normally a drug) that affects the mind. 'Affecting' the mind can simply mean interacting with receptors in the brain to change a mood state or brain chemistry in some way. So if we consider that CBD has been approved as an anti-epilepsy medication and is the subject

of research for mental health conditions such as schizophrenia, PTSD, anxiety and depression, it can be safely assumed that CBD is indeed psychoactive – but in a good way.

However, if you are taking a CBD oil containing more than trace levels of THC (0.2 per cent in the UK or 0.3 per cent in the USA), you may experience some unexpected psychoactive effects. Which is why some people choose a 'broad spectrum' CBD oil, containing zero THC.

But overall, don't expect to feel immediately different after taking CBD oil. For some people this can actually be a bit disappointing.

However, this lack of any mind-altering experiences is a key reason why CBD is non-addictive. In fact, according to current research, CBD may hold potential as a treatment for types of substance abuse, reducing instances of relapse and managing cravings.[16]

CBD VS THC

As the two most abundant cannabinoids in cannabis, CBD and THC will always be intrinsically linked.

For many years, THC was the cannabinoid getting all the column inches (positive and negative) because of its illegality and psychoactive effect. Even within the scientific community, CBD was initially largely ignored and assumed to be inactive.

I like to think of THC and CBD as being two brothers with polar opposite

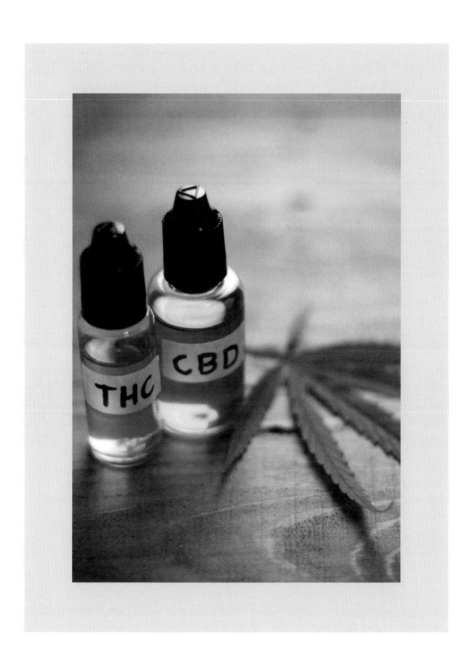

personalities. THC is the wild extrovert, sometimes overpowering in his presence, while CBD is the sensible one who's there to clear up his sibling's mess.

When both compounds are present in cannabis, CBD actually counteracts the high caused by THC. It's one reason why 21st-century black-market cannabis blows the socks off most people. Twenty or thirty years ago, smoking a joint was a more benign, relaxing experience, due to a balanced ratio between the two cannabinoids. These days, recreational tastes demand high THC cannabis strains, so that's what the illegal growers cultivate.

That's not to say that CBD is the 'good' cannabinoid and THC the 'bad' one. This is at best an oversimplification and at worst, completely inaccurate.

THC is already prescribed for chemo-related nausea and vomiting, as well as cachexia (rapid weight loss and muscle wasting) in cancer and HIV patients in countries where medical cannabis is legal. The compound also shows potential as an anti-cancer drug due to its anti-tumoral effects. A further exciting area of research involves combining THC and CBD together as a treatment for cancer, and in conditions such as chronic pain and spasticity in multiple sclerosis.

In the CBD market, many people prefer to use CBD oils containing legally allowed amounts of THC (0.2 per cent in the UK and 0.3 per cent in the US), although opinion remains divided in the UK whether the Home Office actually permits any trace amounts of THC in CBD oil. It's possible a future beckons where only CBD oil with zero THC will be available.

IS CBD OIL THE SAME AS CBD?

While CBD and CBD oil are often used interchangeably, it is important to differentiate between the two.

CBD (cannabidiol) is the molecule, while CBD oil is a hemp (or cannabis) extract containing CBD alongside other compounds found in the plant. After harvesting the hemp, active compounds (including CBD) are extracted using solvents such as carbon dioxide or ethanol. Heat is also applied to turn CBDA into CBD. The sticky hemp paste usually then passes through a filtration process, after which it is mixed with a carrier oil such as hemp seed oil, MCT coconut oil or olive oil.

From a scientific point of view, the average CBD oil available to the public contains a host of 'impurities' (minor cannabinoids, terpenes, flavonoids) and negligible amounts of CBD compared to the amounts administered in clinical trials. That's why you'll often hear scientists dismissing CBD oil as little more than a placebo. And yet, anecdotal reports suggest that whole-plant CBD oil can bring about powerful effects on our health at far lower doses than those used in medical trials and when accompanied by the other molecules found in hemp. Could the millions of people around the world who say CBD oil has helped their health all be wrong?

HOW CBD WORKS

It's no accident that CBD has completely blown apart both the nutritional-supplement and medical-marijuana markets across the globe. Never before has a plant-based health product been used by such an extensive cross section of the population for a whole range of health conditions.

The doubters question whether CBD really can treat everything – pain, anxiety, sleep disorders, epilepsy and potentially even cancer.

However, when you consider the myriad of ways CBD interacts with our bodies, it soon becomes clear that it is no ordinary compound.

CBD THE MULTI-TASKING MOLECULE

A key step in the process of bringing a drug to market is understanding how a substance affects the body.

CBD is considered a pleiotropic molecule, which means it causes diverse effects in our bodies through multiple mechanisms of action.

A key way that compounds create biological reactions is by binding with receptors in our cells. Receptors are like locks, waiting to be opened by chemical keys such as neurotransmitters in order to convert any incoming signals into a biological response.

CBD binds with several different classes of receptors, all of which create very different effects in our body. It's as if CBD were some kind of molecular social butterfly, flitting from one type of receptor to another.

CBD Activates Serotonin Receptors

Many people report feeling happier and less anxious after taking CBD, which scientists believe can be partly explained by its activation of 5-HT1A serotonin receptors in the brain.[17]

Serotonin is a type of neurotransmitter, crucial to maintaining balanced mental wellbeing. Indeed, a widely used class of antidepressant medications act by increasing serotonin signalling.

CBD Binds with Pain Receptors

One of the most common reasons people take CBD is to alleviate pain, and it's thought CBD's activation of the TRPV1 'vanilloid' receptor could be a contributing factor.[18] TRPV1 receptors are found in neurons (nerve cells) involved in pain perception, pain control, inflammation and body temperature.

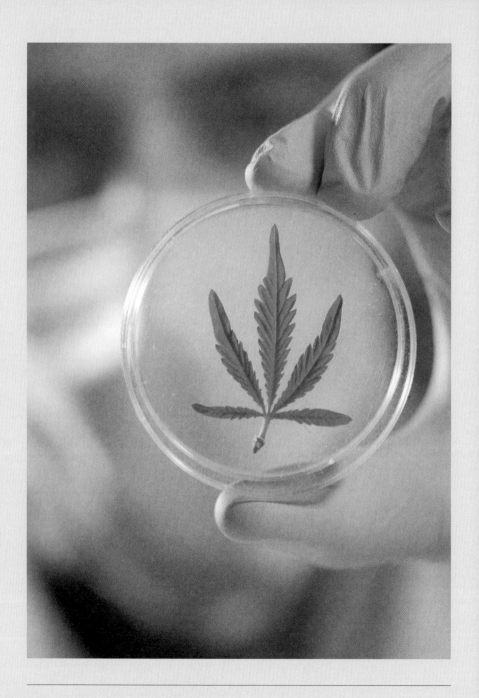

THE CBD BOOK

CBD Activates PPARS Nuclear Receptors

Could CBD be an anti-tumoral drug of the future? The truth is, it's still too early to say, but in preclinical studies scientists have found CBD elicits anti-cancer effects by activating special receptors (peroxisome proliferator activated receptors)[19] that regulate the expression of genes. Not only that, stimulating these receptors may break down amyloid plaque in the brain, the hard clumps of protein that destroy healthy connection between nerve cells in Alzheimer's patients.

CBD Blocks GPR55 Orphan Receptors

Scientists aren't only interested in researching substances that activate receptors. Blocking agents known as antagonists also have a therapeutic place in drug development.

CBD has been found to block GPR55 receptors.[20] An overabundance of these GPR55 receptors has been detected in various types of cancer, and researchers believe their activation may promote the spread of cancer cells.[21] This doesn't mean that CBD cures cancer, but its ability to block GPR55 receptors means it could be an anti-cancer drug of the future.

CBD Modulates the Immune System

Scientists believe CBD elicits its anti-inflammatory effect by suppressing the function of white blood cells called T Cells, reducing the production of pro-inflammatory proteins called cytokines, and stopping inflammatory cells from migrating to other parts of the body.[22]

CBD Is a Powerful Antioxidant

Alongside other cannabinoids, CBD has been found to be a powerful antioxidant, on a par with vitamin C and E.[23] This combined with CBD's overall anti-inflammatory effect and ability to reduce the overproduction of glutamate, a neurotransmitter that can cause brain cell death, means CBD may actually protect our brain cells from age-related damage.

'Its ability to block GPR55 receptors means it could be an anti-cancer drug of the future.'

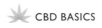

CBD AND THE
ENDOCANNABINOID SYSTEM

Another reason CBD's effects on our health are so wide reaching may be due to the compound's interaction with our endocannabinoid system (ECS).

Don't panic if this is the first time you've heard of the ECS. Despite its discovery in the early 1990s, even most medical schools do not include the ECS in their syllabus.

Why? Well, a clue can be found in the name: endo (meaning within) and cannabinoid (molecules like THC and CBD found in cannabis).

In fact, scientists only discovered the ECS when they were trying to understand THC's psychoactive effects in humans. They found a vast network of receptors named CB1 (CB = for cannabinoid) in our brains and central nervous systems which are directly activated by THC. Another class of receptor (CB2) was later located, predominantly in immune cells. Their activation (again by THC) is thought to have an overall anti-inflammatory effect.

Next, the hunt was on for chemicals produced within the body that bind with the endocannabinoid receptors. With the discovery of the endocannabinoid anandamide, named after the Sanskrit word for bliss, and the less poetic 2-AG, scientists had their answer. However, despite all these amazing breakthroughs, it still wasn't clear what the ECS actually did.

Because endocannabinoids signal backwards across the gaps between neurons, scientists concluded that the ECS must have some kind of modulating function, acting a bit like a dimmer switch – turning up or down cellular activity in order to bring about balance, also known as homeostasis.

Hence the ECS is widely described as a highly dynamic homeostatic regulator, playing an important part in all biological functions; everything from our sleep, appetite, memory, mood, reproduction, immune system, pain control and cell proliferation is regulated by our ECS.

ENDOCANNABINOID DEFICIENCY

We can think of the ECS as the conductor of an orchestra, making sure no one section drowns out another. But what happens when the conductor has an off day or leaves his orchestra unattended? Chaos breaks out and that perfect harmony is lost.

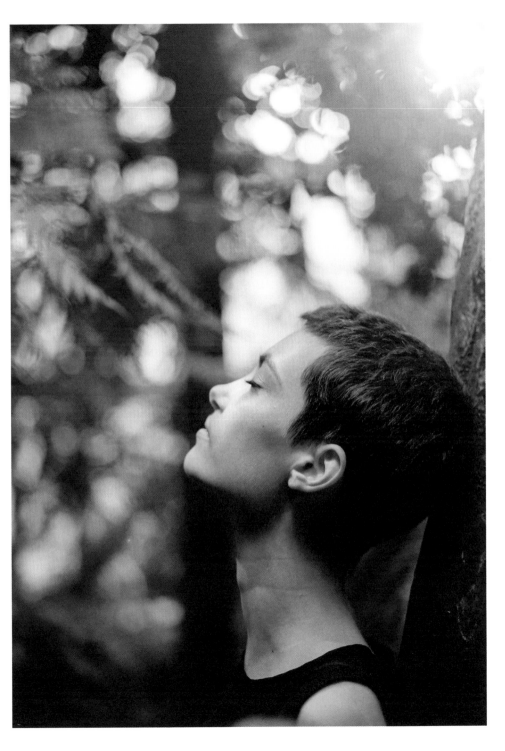

HOW CBD WORKS WITH THE ECS

Unlike THC, CBD does not directly bind with either CB1 or CB2 endocannabinoid receptors. Instead, CBD interacts with the ECS by blocking an enzyme called fatty acid amide hydrolase (FAAH), responsible for breaking anandamide down in the body.

Because endocannabinoids are produced on demand and broken down as soon as their regulating role has been performed, delaying its degradation means anandamide gets to hang out for longer doing its anti-inflammatory, mood-boosting work.

This relationship between CBD, anandamide and FAAH inhibition was highlighted in a clinical trial in which subjects with schizophrenia were given CBD.[26] Researchers noticed that administering CBD appeared to block FAAH, which in turn led to higher anandamide levels, and an overall improvement in psychotic symptoms.

It could also explain why people suffering from conditions falling under the 'endocannabinoid deficiency' umbrella, such as IBS, fibromyalgia and migraines, tend to find their symptoms improve when they are taking CBD.

If your only reason for taking CBD is to support the healthy functioning of your endocannabinoid system, you probably won't be going far wrong.

03

CBD
RESEARCH

A recent study by the Centre for Medical Cannabis, a membership body representing businesses in medical cannabis and the CBD industry, concluded that a 'sizeable proportion' of the 4 to 6 million CBD users in the UK say they experience a medicinal or therapeutic benefit from it.[27] This suggests that as well as taking CBD for overall wellness, many people are using it to treat health conditions, either alongside or instead of prescription medication.

Before taking any medication, be it prescription, over-the-counter or botanical, it's vital to do your own research into any side effects and drug interactions, and most importantly, whether there is sufficient evidence proving its efficacy. These are all questions you should be asking yourself before taking CBD oil for your own health.

Since entering the CBD and medical cannabis industry, I've learned how to pull out the relevant facts from lengthy scientific studies, but this isn't a skill all of us have honed. That's why I've compiled this section on CBD research, kicking off with a quick primer on the truth behind the 'CBD cures X' stories in the newspapers.

Please note, the research listed is correct at the time of writing but additional results from studies may be published subsequently. Even where results are encouraging, they do not constitute sufficient evidence to take CBD instead of your current prescription medication.

OF MICE AND MEN: HOW A DRUG GETS TO MARKET AND WHY IT MATTERS

Unless you're a research scientist or a physician, it's likely you've never spent much time pouring over peer-reviewed academic research papers. The nearest most of us get are the summarised versions used in headline-grabbing articles celebrating the latest cure for cancer. You're not alone if you take these stories at face value. If those clever scientists have proved something in the lab, it must be true in humans, right?

The reality is somewhat different. Discoveries made in petri dishes and tried out on rodents are not necessarily replicated in humans. So, if you're researching CBD for your own health condition, it's vital to know the difference.

ODDS STACKED AGAINST CANNABIS MEDICAL RESEARCH

It's often the case that getting a drug to market is a lengthy process that can take more than a decade and costs billions of pounds. As a result, pharmaceutical companies tend to focus on patentable,

synthetic, single-molecule drugs to be sure they get a decent return on their investment. It's no surprise big pharma has steered clear of whole-plant cannabis and CBD oils, which as botanical extracts containing hundreds of compounds are financial suicide to invest in.

Clinical research has also been stymied by the worldwide Schedule 1 classification deeming cannabis without any medical benefit and liable for abuse.

Professor Manuel Guzmán, Professor of Biochemistry and Molecular Biology at Madrid University and author of several ground-breaking studies into cannabinoids and cancer, describes the barriers faced by researchers.

Doing clinical research with cannabinoids is very complicated because cannabis is controlled by the United Nations and is a Schedule 1 drug, subjected to very strong restrictions in the production, manufacturing, and exporting etc. That means that many clinicians and many investors get frightened. They don't want to get into so much bureaucracy and they prefer to go for substances that are easier to get into clinical trials.

Consequently, in the eyes of health regulators and the medical profession, there is a paucity of evidence proving cannabis (including CBD) is safe and effective in humans. That's not to say there isn't a wide body of observational data and single case studies. But this isn't considered sufficiently reliable by those deciding which medicines we can take.

HOW MUCH CAN WE TRUST PRECLINICAL STUDIES?

Let's take the following story that hit the headlines recently. 'Cannabis Chemical May Help Treat Pancreatic Cancer, Study Finds,' reported one UK broadsheet.[28] The chemical in question was a type of flavonoid (naturally occurring molecules in plants and fruits), which was first tested with promising results on pancreatic cancer cells in test tubes or petri dishes (in vitro).[29] Next step was to extend the investigation to rodents (in vivo) with pancreatic cancer tumours. There's no guarantee that positive in-vitro results are replicated in animals, but in this instance, scientists found the flavonoid slowed both tumour growth and the spread of cancer cells. 'Hurrah', you might think, 'we have a cure for pancreatic cancer.' Well, not exactly. Professor Guzman, who has spent the last 30 years investigating the anti-tumoral properties of cannabinoids, knows very well that mice and men are not the same.

One has to consider when one cures cancer in a mouse, it's not really cancer, it's a model of cancer which has only part of the characteristics of human cancer. So the gap between curing the cancer in a mouse and a human is huge. Even in a sophisticated cancer model in mice – in the end mice are mice. It's not just a 25-gram human. Mice have a much simpler biology than ours. They have a strong capacity for tissue regeneration and a stronger immune system than us. In mice, there are hundreds of molecules that can cure cancer, but there are very few molecules that can do that in humans.

The bottom line is that preclinical trials point towards the therapeutic potential of a substance, and is a vital part of the process of getting a drug to market, but it is only the beginning of the story.

CLINICAL TRIALS

When a pharmaceutical company is confident there's sufficient preclinical evidence showing safety and efficacy of a drug in animals, the next step is to move on to human studies.

Most licensed medicines have been through three phases of randomised clinical trials, which if successfully completed, show they are safe, more effective than a placebo, and give information about appropriate dosing. Randomised controlled trials, the third and final phase in which patients are randomly assigned either the drug being tested, the current standard treatment or a placebo, are considered the gold standard for proving a medicine is safe, effective, and free from patient (or clinician) bias. Without

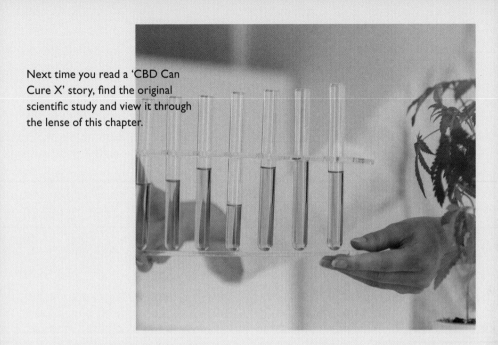

Next time you read a 'CBD Can Cure X' story, find the original scientific study and view it through the lens of this chapter.

this information, doctors do not feel confident prescribing a drug and it will not get recommended by health regulators such as the National Institute for Health and Care Excellence (NICE).

Right now, the only CBD drug to have passed through the three phases of clinical trials has been Epidyolex (purified CBD) for children with Dravet and Lennox-Gastaut Syndromes, two rare types of drug-resistant epilepsy. Phase 2 clinical trials on small numbers of patients are currently taking place, testing CBD

for anxiety, PTSD, schizophrenia, opioid addiction, inflammatory bowel disease, bipolar depression and Parkinson's disease. However, even if these trials are successful, phase 3 studies must be carried out on hundreds or even thousands of patients before CBD can be approved for any of these conditions.

So next time you read a 'CBD Can Cure X' story, find the original scientific study and view it through the lens of this chapter. The same goes for the next section in which I discuss current CBD research.

ADDICTION

A common concern for anyone new to CBD is whether it's possible to become addicted to CBD oil.

Well, as it turns out, CBD is completely non-addictive. It's one of the reasons the World Health Organisation recommended that CBD should not be considered a controlled substance. Not only that, research suggests that CBD may actually help people come off or abstain from addictions to substances such as tobacco, heroin, cocaine and even cannabis itself.

It makes sense if you think about it. Many people develop addictions because they cannot cope with the stresses of their daily life. Then once addicted, coming off a drug is met with horrendous cravings and further anxiety. So a substance that has an anti-anxiety effect could potentially help manage the cravings during the withdrawal period and keep stress at bay during abstinence.

WHAT'S THE EVIDENCE?

Studies on both animals and humans suggest that CBD can indeed reduce cravings in addictions to certain substances.

In one study, heroin addicts were given a single dose of CBD over three consecutive days. They were then exposed to heroin-related and neutral video stimuli at 1 hour, 24 hours and 7 days after the CBD. The subjects receiving CBD had fewer cravings than the placebo group, an effect that lasted for 7 days after treatment.[30]

In everyday terms, this suggests taking CBD when trying to quit an addiction may help to neutralise stimulus that would usually bring about cravings and potential relapse. So if you take CBD, maybe you won't feel like a cigarette so much after that morning coffee.

Or if you're not ready to quit your habit completely, CBD could just be a way to cut down. A double-blind placebo study in which cigarette smokers were encouraged to use an inhaler containing either CBD or a placebo every time they wanted a cigarette, found the CBD group smoked 40 per cent less cigarettes than the placebo group.[31]

Perhaps the most surprising use of CBD in addiction is for the treatment of cannabis dependence itself. Researchers have found that CBD can reduce 'wanting' and 'liking' of cannabis-related stimuli, which basically means it makes smoking weed less enjoyable.[32]

A case history of a 19-year-old with cannabis dependency, suggested CBD can also reduce withdrawal symptoms when quitting cannabis.[33] These findings will hopefully be replicated in the results of a yet-to-be-published clinical trial in which CBD was given to subjects trying to remain abstinent from or become less dependent on cannabis. Researchers hope that improvements in memory, psychological wellbeing, and days in work/education will be noted.[34]

Quitting any addiction is a difficult task. Accessing support through groups such as Alcoholics Anonymous, Narcotics Anonymous or talking to your family doctor are always an advisable first step. However, taking CBD during the process of cutting down or in abstinence could give you the extra help you need to manage the anxiety and any cravings you may experience.

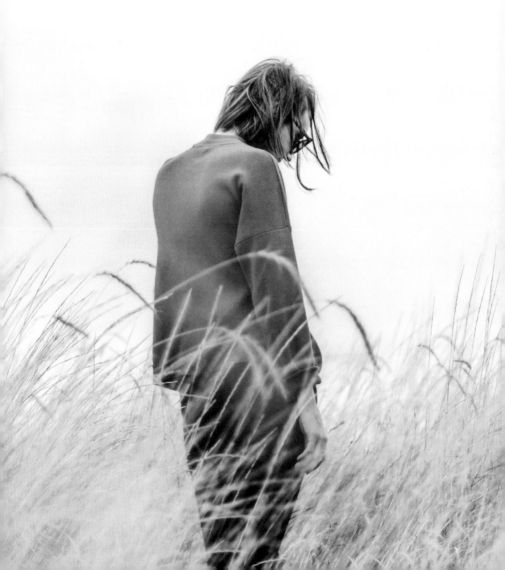

ANXIETY

Combating stress and anxiety is perhaps the most common reason people turn to CBD oil, with one survey in the United States finding that 50 per cent of respondents used CBD oil for stress and anxiety relief.

Even celebrities are getting in on the act with reality TV darling Kim Kardashian claiming CBD oil helped her quit prescription anti-anxiety medication.

Anecdotal accounts are one thing, but how much scientific research actually exists proving CBD oil to be an effective anti-anxiety medication?

HOW CBD CALMS THE MIND

Before getting stuck into the hard evidence, it's worth spending time understanding how CBD affects our mental wellbeing.

Contrary to much of the information out there, CBD is actually a psychoactive substance. You might be thinking, 'Hang on a sec, I was told CBD wasn't going to get me high.' While this is certainly true, 'psychoactive' simply refers to a drug that affects the mind in some way. The fact that taking CBD can cause someone to move from a state of anxiety to a state of calmness, means it is considered to have a psychoactive effect.

How does CBD do this?

Principally, it's through the compound's activation of 5-HT1A serotonin receptor. Serotonin is a type of neurotransmitter that contributes towards good mood and mental wellbeing. By activating the 5-HT1A serotonin receptor, scientists have observed how CBD reduces stress and anxiety in both animals and humans.[35]

Remember the endocannabinoid system (see page 30)? A healthy ECS ensures our fear-based reactions to stimuli don't get out of whack, in turn making us more emotionally resilient. Sometimes, though, our ECS can become dysfunctional, which scientists believe may contribute to the development of anxiety disorders.

Interestingly, in a kind of anxiety-promoting vicious circle, chronic stress can cause a reduction in the number of CB1 endocannabinoid receptors in our brains, while less CB1 receptors contribute directly to anxiety disorders.[36]

How does CBD fit into this?

As mentioned in our chapter on the endocannabinoid system, CBD does not directly bind with the endocannabinoid receptors. Instead, it is thought to increase cell communication by allowing anandamide, the natural cannabis-like molecule named after the Sanskrit word for bliss, to be present in the body for longer. Higher anandamide levels almost certainly contribute to CBD's overall anti-anxiety effect.

WHAT'S THE EVIDENCE?

Very few of us relish the thought of speaking in public, but for someone with social anxiety, it's the ultimate white-knuckle nightmare. So when scientists decided to give subjects with social anxiety CBD before conducting a simulated public speaking test, the results would be a good gauge of whether CBD truly does help reduce anxiety. Encouragingly, administering CBD significantly reduced anxiety, cognitive impairment and discomfort. However, subjects given a placebo weren't so lucky and their anxiety levels shot through the roof.[37]

More recently, similar results were found in a double-blind placebo study targeting young Japanese adults with social anxiety and avoidant personality disorder. They were given 300mg of CBD oil in a single dose each day over 4 weeks, which was subsequently found to significantly reduce their anxiety.[38]

In another study, 72 patients with anxiety and sleep issues were given between 25mg and 75mg of CBD in capsule form alongside their existing treatment. In 79 per cent of the subjects, their anxiety levels dropped and remained reduced for the duration of the study.[39]

While these are positive results indeed, it should be noted that the CBD given in both studies is likely to have been purified CBD and not the full-spectrum CBD oil

commonly available on the high street or online. Plus the dosage – 600mg in the social anxiety study – was far greater than the amount of CBD normally consumed for anxiety, which is somewhere between 10–20mg per day.

However, people who use CBD oil f or anxiety report managing their symptoms with far lower doses.

'Higher anandamide levels almost certainly contribute to CBD's overall anti-anxiety effect.'

AUTISM

Giving CBD or any compound found in cannabis to children can be a controversial subject; however, that is just what is proposed for children with autism spectrum disorder (ASD). At the more severe end of the spectrum children are often given a cocktail of drugs including antipsychotics, antidepressants and anti-seizure medication. However, in some countries where medical cannabis is legal, ASD is considered a qualifying condition, with doctors opting for CBD-dominant strains with reasonable success.

CBD, THE ECS AND AUTISM

Scientists believe compounds like CBD have a therapeutic effect in children with ASD due to their interaction with the body's endocannabinoid system (ECS), which can be dysregulated in autism. Indeed, one study found children with ASD had lower anandamide levels (the natural cannabis-like chemical produced by the body), leading researchers to speculate that one factor contributing to ASD could be a deficient endocannabinoid system.[40] Once again, this could be where CBD comes to the fore due to its ability to strengthen endocannabinoid tone, in particular increasing anandamide signalling.

WHAT'S THE EVIDENCE?

So far, results from two studies have been published showing how CBD positively affects ASD traits in children.[41][42] In both studies, children with ASD were given CBD-rich cannabis oil over a period of months. It's important here to point out that 'CBD-rich' cannabis oil is not the same as hemp CBD oil, as it contains more THC than is legally allowed in most countries. That said, results from both studies were similarly encouraging with considerable improvements experienced in behaviour and communication, as well as quality-of-life criteria such as being able to shower and dress independently.

In one of the studies, 84 per cent of the ASD subjects who also had epilepsy reported 'a disappearance of symptoms' and 33 per cent of children were able to reduce other medication they were taking. A clinical trial has been conducted in Israel using CBD-rich cannabis oil (20:1 CBD:THC) for subjects aged 5 to 21 years with autism, but as yet, results haven't been published.[43]

At some point in the future, CBD may indeed be an approved medication for autism spectrum disorder. However, right now, we're just not there yet. If your child has autism and you are considering giving them CBD oil, make sure you first have a discussion with your doctor.

AUTOIMMUNE DISEASES

'Autoimmune' is an umbrella term used to describe conditions where the immune system attacks the body's own tissues: for example, Hashimoto's disease, multiple sclerosis, Crohn's, lupus, rheumatoid arthritis, type 1 diabetes and ankylosing spondylitis, which are generally treated with immunosuppressant drugs like methotrexate or corticosteroids (steroids). As a rule, steroids should not be prescribed long-term, as they can cause side effects such as high blood pressure, osteoporosis mood swings and weight gain. So researchers are seeking safe and effective ways to mitigate against the effects created in the body by a self-attacking immune system and to treat the symptoms.

WHY CBD?

CBD is widely recognised as having anti-inflammatory effects on the body. For example, we know CBD slows the production of both T-cells (white blood cells which, when dysregulated, can contribute to autoimmune diseases)[44] and cytokines (pro-inflammatory proteins).[45]

CBD's role as a powerful antioxidant also makes it of therapeutic interest in autoimmune diseases where oxidative stress (the imbalance between free radicals and antioxidants in the body) directly contribute to their development.[46]

WHAT'S THE EVIDENCE?

Unfortunately, overall clinical data is rather lacking for the use of CBD as a treatment for autoimmune diseases. One mouse study did show that CBD appeared to improve MS symptoms by decreasing how many T-cells made it into the central nervous system and by reducing levels of pro-inflammatory cytokines.[47] Another found administering CBD reduced inflammation markers in mice with Type 1 diabetes, even delaying the development of the disease.[48] While in a mouse model of myocarditis, an autoimmune-related cause of heart failure in young adults, CBD limited the damage caused to the heart by T-cell infiltration.[49] The authors concluded that 'CBD may represent a promising novel treatment for managing autoimmune myocarditis and possibly other autoimmune disorders and organ transplantation'.

These are promising results in mice, but what about humans? Clinical trials are currently recruiting to see whether CBD could replace the chronic use of steroids in both autoimmune hepatitis[50] and Crohn's disease[51]. It will be interesting to see whether these results reflect the experiences of patients who have been able to reduce or come off long-term steroids after taking CBD oil.

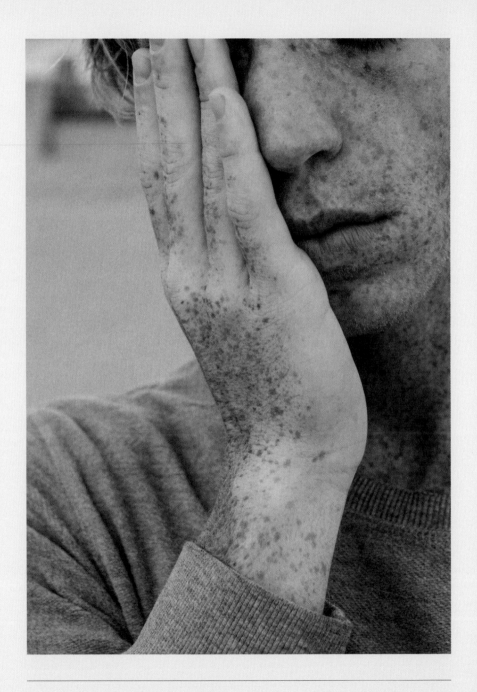

THE CBD BOOK

CANCER

There's a rather large elephant in the room when talking about CBD and our health, and it's whether CBD can treat cancer. If you're reading this book, you've likely seen some of the amazing stories in the media where once-seriously-ill patients attribute their recovery from cancer to CBD. With cancer affecting half of us in our lifetime, it's little surprise so many of us are looking for a wonder cure.

A SINGLE CURE FOR CANCER DOESN'T EXIST

The internet is full of conspiracy stories about how a cure for cancer already exists and has been withheld from the public. But the bottom line is that it's impossible to talk about one cure for cancer, when cancer is actually a collection of illnesses sharing one key factor: for some reason cells in the body forget how to die, continually dividing and growing, until eventually forming a lump or tumour. Often as the tumours grow, cancer cells break off and migrate to other parts of the body, a process known as metastasis.

Not only that, but within each type of cancer there can be different variations. For instance, in breast cancer alone, there are 10 different classifications, all requiring their own unique form of treatment.

So, the likelihood that CBD or indeed any treatment could be a cure for cancer

per se, is unrealistic. That's why any research is performed on a cancer-by-cancer basis, focusing on cancer types where initial preclinical studies have shown promise. The same goes for research into cannabinoids like CBD as a treatment for cancer.

There are some particular types of cancer, such as glioblastoma, an aggressive and difficult-to-treat form of brain tumour, where research has advanced further. By this, I mean scientists have moved beyond studying cancer cells in petri dishes or animal models, to clinical trials in humans.

CBD SHOWS ANTI-CANCER POTENTIAL (JUST DON'T GET TOO EXCITED YET)

So far, any clinical trials using cannabinoids have involved THC, the psychoactive and illegal compounds in cannabis, or a combination of THC and CBD. However, for many years, CBD's non-intoxicating effect meant it was believed to be without sufficient therapeutic punch for a disease like cancer.

But as scientists gain more knowledge about how CBD affects the body, they've realised the complex mechanisms by which the compound affects the body may actually create an anti-cancer effect.

Take, for instance, CBD's deactivation of the GPR55 orphan receptor, thought to be a potential third endocannabinoid receptor. Increased GPR55 activity has been found in certain types of cancer and is thought to promote the reproduction of cancer cells and increased tumour burden (the number of cancer cells, the size of a tumour or the amount of cancer in the body).[52] So finding a way to block this signalling could have anti-cancer effects. Which is where CBD comes in. CBD is considered a GPR55 antagonist; instead of binding with the receptor, it inhibits it. Could this mechanism give CBD anti-tumoral effects? Well, that's what researchers are trying to find out in their labs.

That's not the end of CBD's anti-cancer potential. CBD's activation of peroxisome proliferator-activated receptors, a class of receptor located on the cell's nucleus, may cause cancer cell death and tumour regression in lung cancer.[53]

But before we all get too over-excited about CBD being the latest cancer cure, these studies offer no proof of their anti-cancer effects in patients, they just point towards the biological mechanisms by which this might happen.

WHAT'S THE EVIDENCE?

There's a reason why millions of pounds are being spent around the world researching whether CBD could be an anti-cancer drug. Scientists have observed how, in preclinical studies at least, CBD ticks many of the boxes necessary for a successful cancer treatment.

1. CBD Kills Cancer Cells

Cell death (apoptosis) is part of life. But for some reason, cancer cells appear to ignore the messages from the body telling them to die. Instead the cells keep dividing, growing and spreading, wreaking havoc around the body.

THC, cannabis' psychoactive compound, was the first cannabinoid found to activate cell suicide in cancer cells. But what about CBD? A number of preclinical studies have shown CBD's cancer-killing effect in action. In one breast cancer preclinical study, CBD caused oestrogen-receptor-positive and oestrogen-receptor-negative breast cancer cell death, while keeping healthy cells intact.[54] Another found combining CBD with radiotherapy in leukaemia brought about apoptosis in leukaemia cells, while not affecting non-cancerous white blood cells.[55] CBD also killed cancer cells in some preclinical studies for neuroblastoma, an aggressive and difficult-to-treat class of brain cancer.[56]

2. CBD Stops Tumours from Growing

As well as killing cancer cells, scientists are interested in both limiting the growth of tumours and preventing them from invading healthy surrounding tissue.

Again, CBD shows some initial promise. A 2006 breast cancer study found CBD hindered growth in some breast cancer cell lines.[57] CBD also inhibits the ID1 gene, which when dysregulated can lead to breast cancer cells spreading.[58] Scientists have also noted how CBD can cut off a tumour's blood supply, limiting its ability to grow and spread.[59] It's fair to say, then, that based on current preclinical evidence, CBD shows promise as a treatment for cancer.

A LACK OF CLINICAL EVIDENCE

But, and there is a but, right now there is an absence of clinical trials for CBD as an anti-cancer treatment for all the reasons previously mentioned.

In 2018, a case series was published reporting the results from 119 patients treated with synthetic CBD on a 'three days on, three days off' basis over a period of four years.[60] According to the paper's author, clinical responses were seen in 92 per cent of the 199 patients, which included reductions in both circulating tumour cells and tumour size. The report mentions in particular the case of a five-year-old boy with anaplastic ependymoma, a rare brain tumour, who prior to starting CBD had exhausted all treatment options. Ten months after beginning his CBD treatment, a scan revealed the boy's tumour had shrunk by 60 per cent.

CBD AND CHEMO – BETTER TOGETHER?

As compelling as this evidence may seem, it is unlikely that CBD will ever be approved as a standalone anticancer treatment. However, it is quite possible clinical trials will take place for CBD as an 'add on' treatment or adjuvant to existing cancer therapy.

Dr Wai Liu, Research Fellow at St Georges in London and author of this book's foreword, has witnessed in his own lab, how combining CBD with chemotherapy can lead to enhanced anticancer activity in preclinical studies.[61] Dr Liu explains:

CBD is a chemical that has been shown to exhibit anticancer properties in laboratory and animal studies. The mechanisms of action are complex, but are associated with modifications to intracellular signalling pathways that underpin cell functions such as growth and death. Studies have also shown that changes to these pathways can prime some cancer cells to the actions of other treatments.

For instance, as CBD is capable of increasing the expression of cellular proteins required for death to occur in some cancer cells, using it before other treatments can be beneficial, as the cancer cells would have been set up to die in response to other treatment. This is how I see a future for CBD, as an adjuvant therapy that supports and bolsters the action of other treatments such as chemotherapy and radiotherapy.

Indeed, the only phase 2 clinical trials currently taking place for cannabinoids and cancer (a combination of THC and CBD for patients with glioblastoma) are examining whether THC/CBD plus chemotherapy is more effective than chemotherapy alone.[62]

SHOULD PATIENTS TAKE CBD FOR CANCER? A SCIENTIST'S VIEW

As a medical cannabis journalist, I've been in the fortunate position to interview a number of scientists specialising in researching cannabis as a treatment for cancer over the years.

They are without exception an incredibly cautious bunch, because despite what you might have read on the internet, it's still not possible to say that cannabis, CBD or indeed any of the cannabinoids can cure cancer. At best, they will acknowledge that, yes, in certain people and in certain types of cancer, cannabis shows promising anticancer activity.

Dr Liu is himself regularly contacted by patients who report positive results after taking CBD oil for their cancer, but still maintains that until we know more, patients should exhaust all 'conventional' options before starting CBD.

In some situations CBD can actually alter the activity of other drugs. Not only can CBD antagonise a drug directly by altering the signalling pathways that control cell fate in cancer cells, but in some cases because it is metabolised by certain organs in the body, these organs can be hyperactivated and end up changing the activity of other drugs that may be being used at the same time. That's not to say the effects are always negative because we've shown positive synergies. However, it's sensible to ensure the drugs being given by the doctor are given every opportunity to work.

We're talking about a drug, a chemotherapy that's proven to work; it has gone through all the clinical trials. From a statistical perspective it seems to work well. So why would you want to jeopardise its action by using a drug such as CBD, which you think works but you haven't got the proof?

Dr Liu does, however, think taking CBD in the gap between cancer diagnosis and the commencement of treatment could be a prudent option.

I think the general idea of utilising something such as CBD in that period of time between diagnosis and 'formal' treatment such as surgery is sensible. Some people have thought about doing this, as they are worried that nothing is happening therapeutically during that window. Whether or not this approach is useful has yet to be determined; however, as long as CBD does not impact the planned surgery, then intuitively it should be a consideration.

When diagnosed with cancer, making decisions about treatment options is ultimately down to the individual. That said, patients are usually encouraged by their oncologist to follow the statistically most efficacious route for their particular type and stage of cancer. If you do decide to incorporate CBD oil into your treatment programme, be sure to discuss this with your specialist so that they can monitor any changes that may occur.

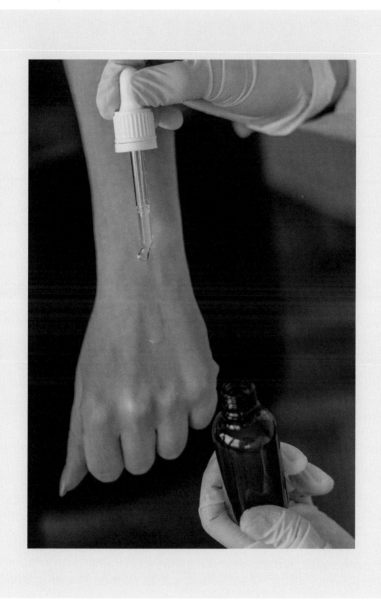

CHRONIC PAIN

Chronic pain is one of the most common reasons people turn to CBD oil.

In the UK, a fifth of the population struggle with chronic pain – that's a whopping 28 million adults. Many patients find the medication offered by their doctor either ineffective at managing their pain, or too laden with unwanted side effects. Chronic pain almost always negatively impacts on quality of life, with many patients experiencing sleep disturbance and low mood.

It's little wonder that any product promising to make life a bit less painful quickly raises hope among the chronic pain community.

WHAT'S THE EVIDENCE?

Unfortunately, very little clinical evidence exists proving CBD's efficacy for chronic pain. Consequently, the likes of the National Institute for Health and Care Excellence (NICE) does not recommend NHS doctors prescribe CBD for chronic pain.

However, many patients taking over-the-counter CBD oil for their chronic pain condition report some improvement both in pain and quality of life. This is echoed in the results of a survey conducted by Project CBD, a US-based not-for-profit medical cannabis educational site. Of the 3,506 people surveyed, 2,202 reported using CBD oil for pain. Of these, 90 per cent found improvements in the frequency and duration after taking CBD oil, and 60 per cent said CBD made their pain much better.[63]

For the purpose of this book, I discuss two pain-related pathologies: arthritis (see page 52) and fibromyalgia (see opposite), but this doesn't mean CBD oil won't potentially provide relief for other diseases associated with chronic pain. Other chronic pain-related conditions, such as IBS, inflammatory bowel disease (see page 60) and autoimmune conditions will be dealt with separately.

> '2,202 reported using CBD oil for pain. Of these, 90 per cent of these found improvements in the frequency and duration after taking CBD oil, and 60 per cent said CBD made their pain much better.'

FIBROMYALGIA

Of all chronic pain sufferers, it's perhaps those with fibromyalgia who are CBD's biggest advocates. As well as the intense, often burning pain, fibro patients tend to experience extreme fatigue, low mood and anxiety.

When one considers that fibromyalgia is one of the most likely contenders in the group of illnesses caused by endocannabinoid deficiency, it becomes less of a surprise that patients report such great improvements when taking CBD oil.

Our endocannabinoid system (ECS) comprises receptors throughout our brain, central nervous system, organs and immune system that are activated by cannabis-like chemicals called endocannabinoids (anandamide and 2-AG) and bring about balance in our bodies and minds.

So if we're experiencing pain for no obvious reason, it's likely our ECS isn't doing its job effectively and may need a little additional help.

This is potentially where CBD comes in. We know that CBD indirectly boosts anandamide levels by blocking the enzyme that breaks it down in the body. So, it's theorised that by taking CBD we can improve our 'endocannabinoid tone', bringing a deficient ECS back into balance again and improving the symptoms associated with endocannabinoid deficiency.

While this causal relationship between endocannabinoid deficiency and fibromyalgia still remains a theory, CBD's anti-inflammatory, analgesic and anti-anxiety effects means the compound shows unique potential as a fibromyalgia drug of the future.

WHAT'S THE EVIDENCE?

A number of observational studies have been conducted, examining the safety and efficacy of medical cannabis (containing both THC and CBD) for fibromyalgia, but none using CBD oil alone.

The most recent study, published in 2019, found that in over 80 per cent of fibromyalgia patients, their pain levels halved after taking medical cannabis over six months.[64]

That said, the 2019 NICE guidelines on medical cannabis called for more research exploring the clinical and cost-effectiveness of CBD as a potential alternative to existing medication for fibromyalgia, which often causes side effects such as nausea, drowsiness and mood disturbance.[65]

ARTHRITIS

Treating the pain associated with arthritis is an often-cited reason for turning to CBD. Hardly surprising when you consider arthritis is the number one cause of disability in older adults. Anecdotal reports abound celebrating CBD's seemingly miraculous pain-relieving effects; however, robust scientific evidence is scant.

Arthritis can be broadly split into two categories:

1. Osteoarthritis (OA)

The degeneration of cartilage in joints due to wear and tear

2. Rheumatoid arthritis (RA)

A class of autoimmune disease whereby the body's immune system attacks the joints.

Both OA and RA are characterised by musculoskeletal pain and inflammation. Patients with OA might also experience neuropathic pain caused by pinched nerves.

Depending on the level of severity, patients are usually prescribed over-the-counter pain relief such as paracetamol or non-steroidal anti-inflammatory drugs (NSAIDS) like ibuprofen or aspirin. In OA, as affected joints further degenerate, patients may be given drugs like gabapentin or even opioids such as tramadol. RA patients are also often prescribed immunosuppressants like methotrexate, a class of chemotherapy drug, in a bid to keep the immune system under control.

Despite this veritable cocktail of pain meds, many arthritis sufferers continue to live with unbearable pain. Little wonder finding a more natural, side-effect-free alternative is an attractive prospect.

CBD AND ARTHRITIS

The fact that CBD relieves pain and has anti-inflammatory properties makes it an ideal candidate for a potential arthritis drug of the future. For patients with RA, CBD's immunoregulation may help curb the destruction caused by an overzealous immune system. Anecdotal reports are certainly favourable, but like any drug, CBD works for some, while not so much for others.

At the very least, taking CBD may mean patients can reduce their other pain medication, minimising their pill burden and resulting side effects. However, any changes should be overseen by a health professional.

WHAT'S THE EVIDENCE?

Again, right now positive patient testimonies currently outweigh hard scientific evidence.

Studies on rats with OA show CBD's anti-inflammatory effect prevented pain and nerve damage.[66, 67] Another rodent study found CBD applied topically as a gel reduced joint pain and swelling.[68]

Encouragingly, a recent randomised placebo study in which patients with peripheral neuropathy topically applied

CBD, found CBD application caused a 'statistically significant reduction in intense pain, sharp pain, cold and itchy sensations' compared to the placebo.[69]

Hopefully, the next few years will bring further results from studies proving CBD really is effective for managing the pain associated with arthritis.

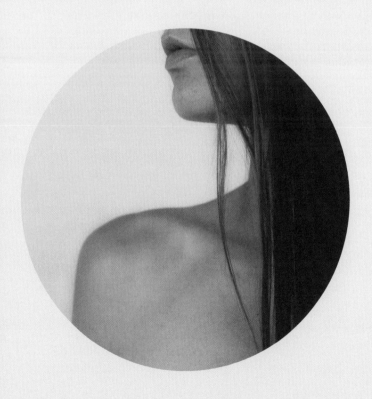

CORONAVIRUS

I started writing this book in the 'pre-coronavirus era' – you remember those days when we were free to travel, shop when we wanted, go to the pub/yoga/choir/football practice (insert your own group activity of choice here), and generally lived without fear of falling victim to one of the most contagious viruses of the last century. But here we are now in the midst of a pandemic, united by social isolation and our cupboards stockpiled with tinned tomatoes and pasta.

Covid-19, the disease resulting from infection by the coronavirus, is of course no joking matter and in a small percentage of cases can be fatal. Thankfully, most of us are hardwired to fight off outside invaders like viruses, thanks to our immune system: the complex network of cells, tissues and organs that runs with military precision to keep us healthy.

There are all sorts of things we can do to support immune function: sleeping well, eating plenty of fresh fruit and vegetables, exercising and managing our stress levels. Who hasn't come down with a cold or flu in the winter months after burning the candle at both ends, drinking too much booze or eating junk food (or all of the above)?

However, with the panic and anxiety surrounding the coronavirus, many of us are looking at ways to bring in some 'immune-boosting big guns', so that our bodies become Teflon to the virus. Only our immune system doesn't really operate in that way.

Unfortunately, that's not stopping a few unscrupulous CBD companies suggesting CBD oil can either boost the immune system or protect us from catching the virus – which is, I'm afraid, a false claim.

CBD AND THE IMMUNE SYSTEM

That's not to say that CBD has no effect on the immune system. Because CBD is anti-inflammatory, it has been surmised that CBD has an overall immunosuppressant or possible immunomodulating effect in the body.[70]

Inflammation tends to get a bad rap, but it is in fact produced by the immune system in response to outside invaders just like viruses, and it initiates the healing process. So, not such a bad guy after all.

However, when this inflammation occurs on a chronic basis or as the result of an overactive immune system, tissue and organ damage can occur. That's why many patients with autoimmune diseases such as rheumatoid arthritis and Crohn's disease, report an improvement in symptoms when taking CBD because it actually dampens down a heightened immune response.

What does this mean for CBD and the coronavirus? Current advice suggests avoiding anti-inflammatory drugs like ibuprofen when we start showing signs of Covid-19, as reducing the inflammation could hamper the immune response, making it harder to get over the disease.[71] Could the same rule be applied to CBD? The truth is, we still don't know.

However, as scientists learn more about the virus, it is becoming clear that when patients are in the latter, more severe stages of the disease, their immune systems have moved into a hyper-inflammatory state, causing what's known as a cytokine storm.[72]

Cytokines are protein messengers secreted by immune cells that increase or decrease inflammation. For reasons yet to be understood, in a small number of patients there is an overproduction of pro-inflammatory cytokines causing the lung damage and respiratory issues associated with the latter stage of Covid-19. As such, patients are given immunosuppressants like corticosteroids to limit the lung damage caused by the hyper-inflammation.

Because CBD is considered anti-inflammatory and even being investigated as a possible alternative to steroids in autoimmune diseases, there may be a time when CBD could be used to suppress the immune system in Covid-19. However, the data just isn't there yet.

The bottom line is that right now, it's best to stick to a 'precautionary approach' – that is, until scientific research and patient data tells us definitively that CBD is an appropriate and safe treatment in Covid-19, we should proceed with caution and follow doctors' advice.

'There may be a time when CBD could be used to suppress the immune system in Covid-19. However, the data just isn't there yet.'

DEPRESSION

Treating depression is one of the most popular reasons people turn to CBD oil. A quarter of us will experience depression at some time in our lives. For those with moderate to heavy depression, antidepressants may be necessary, while for mild depression, talking therapy and even exercise can improve symptoms.

Selective serotonin reuptake inhibitors (SSRIs) are a commonly prescribed class of antidepressants. As with anxiety, the fact that CBD activates 5-HT1A serotonin receptors has led scientists to believe CBD may also have antidepressant effects. Not only that, dysregulation in the endocannabinoid system has been noted in patients in depressed states.[73]

In one curious study, people with a genetic mutation causing them to produce less FAAH (fatty acid amide hydrolase – responsible for breaking down the 'joy molecule' anandamide) were more emotionally resilient and less anxious.[74]

More anandamide in our bodies generally leads to better mood and may be one reason why doing sport is as effective for mild depression as antidepressants. Scientists now know that when we do strenuous cardiovascular exercise, anandamide levels increase.[75] It's thought that the 'runner's high' most of us have had at some point in our lives, is as much to do with anandamide as endorphins.

It's possible, then, that CBD's FAAH inhibition and resultant increases in anandamide may explain why many people say taking CBD oil has helped with their depression.

WHAT'S THE EVIDENCE?

Right now, most studies for CBD and depression have been at the preclinical level. Considering the complexity of depression, we should be cautious about extrapolating too much from any successes in unhappy rodents.

That said, administering CBD to Wistar-Kyoto rats, who naturally exhibit depressive-like symptoms, seemed to make them happier, improving their curiosity and motivation.[76]

Unfortunately, at the time of writing, there have been no completed clinical trials for CBD in depression. One phase 2/3 double-blind placebo trial for CBD as an adjunctive drug for bipolar depression is currently recruiting in Brazil. However, the results are not expected until 2021.

This lack of clinical data proving CBD's efficacy as an antidepressant means that right now there's not enough evidence to suggest it is safe to take CBD instead of a prescribed antidepressant. Please do not stop or reduce your medication without discussing it first with your doctor.

EPILEPSY

Hearing about CBD's ability to reduce seizures in children was the first time many people heard about its therapeutic potential. Since Charlotte Figi's story first hit the media, countless other children have experienced fewer seizures after taking CBD oil.

What's even more striking is that there's often no difference between the CBD oil taken by children like Charlotte and that used as a wellness product.

To be clear, I'm not referring here to Epidyolex, the purified CBD pharmaceutical drug approved in the US and Europe. Nor the high-profile cases of children like Alfie Dingley and Billy Caldwell, whose seizures were only fully controlled when combining THC with CBD oil.

But all around the world, children (and adults) are benefitting from the anticonvulsant effects of just the kind of CBD you or I can buy on the high street or online. Which makes CBD oil a pretty unique botanical product.

Scientists still aren't completely sure why CBD appears to be such a game changer for many epilepsy patients. They suspect CBD's 5-HT1A serotonin receptor activation may be one factor, alongside an overall neuroprotective effect, and its interaction with the body's endocannabinoid system.

WHAT'S THE EVIDENCE?

It's fair to say there's indisputable evidence that CBD, the compound, has anticonvulsant effects in epilepsy. That's why GW Pharma has spent billions of dollars developing Epidyolex, a pure CBD epilepsy drug that reduces seizures by approximately 40 per cent.

Right now, Epidyolex has only been approved for the two rare childhood epileptic conditions Dravet and Lennox-Gastaut syndromes, neither of which respond to conventional anti-epilepsy drugs.

Clinical trials are currently underway testing Epidyolex on other types of epilepsy, but currently in the UK it cannot be prescribed on the NHS for anything other than Dravet and Lennox-Gastaut.

But what about the types of whole-plant CBD oils taken by children like Charlotte Figi?

In 2018, a meta-analysis combining results from multiple scientific studies compared the efficacy of purified CBD products (like Epidyolex) and 'CBD-rich' extracts – cannabis oils containing high levels of CBD.[77] The CBD-rich extracts improved seizures in 71 per cent of cases, compared to 46 per cent of those using purified CBD.

The bottom line is that if you are considering taking CBD alongside your or your child's anti-epilepsy drugs, you should first discuss any possible interactions with your doctor or neurologist.

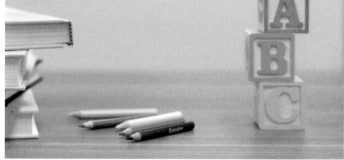

Patients taking CBD-rich extracts took significantly less CBD on average: 6mg of CBD per kilo of body weight a day, compared with 25.3mg of the purified CBD. These higher doses may explain why patients taking purified CBD reported more side effects than the CBD-rich extract group.

While the results do provide a striking argument for using whole-plant CBD-rich oils, it is important to point out that there are no 'quality' randomised clinical trials for CBD-rich extracts. For that reason, doctors in the NHS will not prescribe CBD oil to treat epilepsy.

A NOTE OF CAUTION

In the Epidyolex clinical trials, CBD was administered to children alongside existing anti-epilepsy drugs they were taking. It soon became apparent that CBD was causing

levels of one particular anti-epilepsy drug, Clobazam, to increase in the bloodstream.[78]

Why does this matter? An important part of clinical trials is to work out the optimum dose needed for a drug to be effective with minimal side effects. Key to this is understanding how much of a medication is broken down and excreted, and how much is utilised by the body.

In this case, CBD appeared to increase how much Clobazam was absorbed by the body, resulting in heightened side effects. However, as soon as this was detected, doctors reduced patients' anti-seizure medication, and the side effects abated.

So the bottom line is that if you are considering taking CBD alongside you or your child's anti-epilepsy drugs, you should first discuss any possible interactions with your doctor or neurologist.

HEART DISEASE AND

HYPERTENSION

Taking CBD to protect our hearts against cardiovascular disease is one of the lesser-known potential health benefits of the cannabis compound.

I've heard a few patients mention how since taking CBD oil for a completely unrelated condition, their hypertension has improved and they've been able to reduce their blood pressure medication. Anecdotal evidence, of course, but interesting nonetheless.

Preclinical studies on animal models suggest that because CBD is a powerful antioxidant and has an anti-inflammatory effect, it may protect patients' hearts against the damage caused by diabetes[79] and even heart attacks.[80]

WHAT'S THE EVIDENCE?

Unfortunately, very little human clinical data is available to say whether CBD has any therapeutic effect in heart disease. However, the hypothesis that CBD may reduce blood pressure in times of stress has been examined with promising results.

A study from Nottingham University showed how administering a single dose of 600mg CBD to healthy subjects before exposure to stress not only lowered resting blood pressure, but resulted in lower blood pressure after stress exposure compared to the placebo group.[81]

In a recently published paper, the same CBD dose repeatedly administered to healthy subjects over seven days not only lowered blood pressure during stress, but also reduced arterial stiffness and improved heart function.[82]

From this, it could be extrapolated that taking CBD could protect us from the damaging effects to our hearts caused by stress-related high blood pressure. However, it must be noted that in this study, healthy patients were given 600mg of purified CBD in a single dose, which is approximately the same amount of CBD found in an entire bottle of over-the-counter CBD oil.

At the time of writing, no clinical research has taken place testing CBD's therapeutic benefits on patients with heart disease, although a future Mexican non-placebo study will see whether CBD is safe and well tolerated in patients with heart failure.[83]

IBS AND INFLAMMATORY

BOWEL DISEASE

Irritable Bowel Syndrome (IBS) and Inflammatory Bowel Disease (IBD) are two classes of conditions affecting the bowel and digestive tract, where sufferers experience abdominal pain, inflammation and constipation/diarrhoea.

Patients have been known to successfully manage their symptoms by using CBD oil and/or cannabis oil that contains THC.

IRRITABLE BOWEL SYNDROME (IBS)

IBS is the most common type of gastrointestinal disorder, affecting 10 to 15 per cent of the population. Episodes can be brought on by stress, intolerances to certain types of food and hormonal fluctuations.

IBS has also been linked to endocannabinoid deficiency. Indeed, patients who experience conditions associated with endocannabinoid deficiency, such as fibromyalgia, chronic fatigue and migraines, also tend to have IBS.

At present, there's more anecdotal evidence than clinical studies suggesting CBD has therapeutic benefits for IBS, but the fact that CBD helps manage stress and anxiety, as well as being anti-inflammatory, may explain why IBS sufferers report getting some relief.

INFLAMMATORY BOWEL DISEASE (IBD)

Inflammatory Bowel Disease (which includes Crohn's disease and ulcerative colitis), is an umbrella term to describe disorders caused by inflammation in the gut.

Symptoms tend to be more severe than IBS, and also include weight loss, fever and fatigue and blood in the stools, with many sufferers requiring several surgeries to remove affected parts of the digestive tract.

Excess inflammation, a sign of an overactive immune system, lies at the root of both diseases, while ulcerative colitis itself is actually classed as an autoimmune condition because the body is attacking its own tissues.

As a result, standard treatment involves anti-inflammatory drugs such as corticosteroids or immunosuppressants, which often come with difficult-to-tolerate side effects.

That's why many IBD patients have turned to compounds within the cannabis plant that have both anti-inflammatory and pain-relieving properties.

The ability of cannabinoids to bring the endocannabinoid system back into balance, which often becomes altered in

THE CBD BOOK

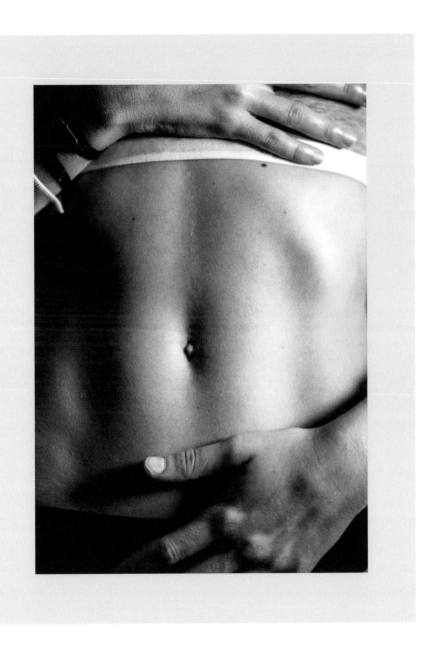

IBD patients, may also explain their therapeutic effect.[84]

WHAT'S THE EVIDENCE?

Most research into cannabinoids and IBD has focused on cannabis containing THC, as this is what's most frequently used by patients. However, preliminary studies suggest CBD has a protective effect in the presence of intestinal inflammation, as well as helping to maintain a healthy intestinal barrier.[85]

One study on 46 subjects with Crohn's disease, found a CBD-dominant cannabis oil (15 per cent CBD oil: 4 per cent THC) brought about a significant improvement in disease symptoms and overall quality of life. After 2 months of treatment, 65 per cent of the cannabis-oil group met the criteria for a full remission of Crohn's symptoms, compared to 35 per cent of the placebo group.[86]

Scientists assumed the cannabinoids' anti-inflammatory effect brought about the overall improvement in symptoms, but this assumption was turned upside down when no significant alterations in inflammation markers were found.

It's important to note that the THC levels used in this study were way above the amounts available in over-the-counter CBD oils, and would therefore be classed as a medical cannabis and not a wellness product.

However, a number of clinical trials are taking place using purified CBD either as a standalone treatment for IBD[87] or to see whether CBD could be a steroid-sparing therapy in steroid-dependent Crohn's patients.[88]

Again, the CBD used in these trials is not comparable to your average CBD oil bought online or on the high street. But the studies do at least show how CBD, the compound, may bring relief to IBD patients in the future.

'After 2 months of treatment, 65 per cent of the cannabis-oil group met the criteria for a full remission of Crohn's symptoms, compared to 35 per cent of the placebo group.'

NEURODEGENERATIVE

DISEASES

In the Western world we are living longer, but as our life expectancy increases, so does our chances of getting neurodegenerative diseases such as dementia or Parkinson's.

That's because as our brains age, they can experience toxic build-up, inflammation and damage through oxidative stress, making us more susceptible to neurodegenerative diseases.

New medication is being developed to improve symptoms like psychosis and motor problems, or to slow down disease progression itself. In the latter category, researchers are searching for drugs that are antioxidant, anti-inflammatory and reduce the damage caused by toxic chemicals in the brain. Guess what: cannabinoids like CBD appear to hit all three targets.

That's why the US Government took out a patent back in 2003 on CBD as an antioxidant and neuroprotectant, stating: 'Cannabinoids are found to have particular application as neuroprotectants, for example in limiting neurological damage following ischemic insults, such as stroke and trauma, or in the treatment of neurodegenerative diseases, such as Alzheimer's disease, Parkinson's disease and HIV dementia.'[89]

The patent highlights CBD's potential, saying, 'Non-psychoactive cannabinoids, such as cannabidiol, are particularly advantageous to use because they avoid toxicity that is encountered with psychoactive cannabinoids at high doses useful in the method of the present invention.'

THE ENDOCANNABINOID SYSTEM AND NEURODEGENERATIVE DISEASES

So, remember the endocannabinoid system (ECS), the vast network of receptors activated by cannabis-like chemicals called endocannabinoids? Turns out the CB1 endocannabinoid receptors are the most abundant class of receptors in our brains and central nervous system. Indeed, the ECS itself modulates neurotransmission, oxidative stress, and the production of proteins, all of which become dysregulated in neurodegenerative diseases.

It should also be noted that some ECS dysregulation can be found in all neurodegenerative diseases. However, we just don't know whether this is the ECS trying to bring the body back into balance again, or whether it's contributing directly to the diseases themselves. Because cannabinoids like CBD interact with the endocannabinoid system, scientists believe they show exciting potential in treating neurodegenerative diseases.[90]

WHAT'S THE EVIDENCE?

Alzheimer's

Dementia, which includes Alzheimer's, is the most common form of neurodegenerative disease, affecting one in three of us in our lifetime.

Unfortunately, there isn't enough evidence right now to suggest CBD has a therapeutic effect on dementia or Alzheimer's, although a preclinical study showed CBD reduced neural inflammation in mice injected with amyloid-β (Aβ), the protein scientists believe leads to brain cell death in Alzheimer's.[91]

However, a small pilot study will be taking place to see whether giving between 20 to 40mg of CBD daily improves behavioural symptoms in adults with Alzheimer's. But we are a long way off CBD being considered an effective drug for dementia.[92]

Parkinson's

The relationship between Parkinson's and the cannabis plant has been cemented ever since some jaw-dropping videos surfaced on the internet in which Parkinson's patients' tremors were seen to miraculously disappear after cannabis was consumed.

In all likelihood, these patients had consumed cannabis containing THC, which by activating CB1 receptors in the brain and central nervous system had brought the tremors to a halt.

But that doesn't mean CBD is without positive effects on other lesser-known Parkinson's symptoms such as psychosis[93] and rapid eye movement sleep behaviour disorder[94], both of which improved in studies when Parkinson's patients were given CBD.

Indeed, a phase 1 clinical trial is currently taking place at King's College, London to see whether CBD can treat the hallucinations and delusions sometimes experienced by Parkinson's patients, while a phase 2 trial in the United States will focus on CBD and Parkinson's motor symptoms. [95, 96]

It's not uncommon for patients with Parkinson's to experience anxiety; however, stress tends to worsen tremor severity. In a recent randomised clinical trial, 24 Parkinson's patients were given 300mg of CBD before performing a simulated public speaking test. Not only were their tremors less pronounced during the stress test compared to the placebo group, but their overall anxiety was reduced.[97]

Multiple Sclerosis

Until recently, MS was the only condition in the UK that could legally be treated with a cannabis-based medication. Sativex, containing equal proportions of THC and CBD, has successfully passed through the three phases of double-blind placebo studies required to bring a drug to market.

Consequently, as all MS clinical studies so far have combined both THC and CBD, there are no human MS studies testing just CBD. However, because MS is classified as an autoimmune disease, CBD's immunoregulatory action could have some therapeutic benefit; a hypothesis proven in a mouse model of MS.[98] Where does this leave you if you have a neurodegenerative disease and are considering CBD oil? As always, it's important to discuss with your doctor whether CBD could negatively interact with your current medication. Thankfully, compared to five years ago, many more physicians have at least a rudimentary knowledge of cannabinoids, so they might be less shocked by the idea of taking CBD oil than you imagine.

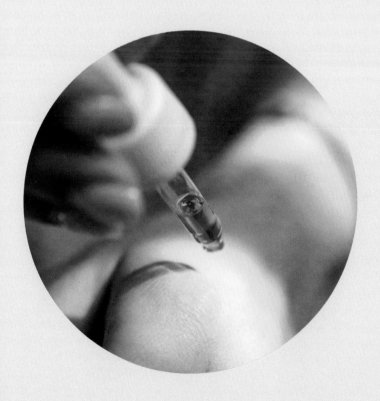

PSYCHOSIS

Cannabis and psychosis have been linked over the years, but for all the wrong reasons. Heavy or long-term cannabis use is thought to increase the likelihood of schizophrenia or psychosis in individuals with a family history of the disease. How could it be then that a compound found in cannabis could also be a potential antipsychotic drug?

CBD as a treatment for psychosis in schizophrenia and other types of mental illness, is one of the few areas where several clinical trials have taken place. Results so far are promising, particularly when CBD is used in conjunction with other existing antipsychotic medications.

Before proceeding any further, it is important to point out that clinical research is still at a preliminary stage, and until a CBD-based antipsychotic drug has been approved by a regulatory body such as the FDA or MHRA, patients should not make any changes to their existing medication.

It should also be noted that purified CBD was used at high doses in the clinical studies, and not whole-plant extracts like those available over the counter or online.

THE CBD, ANANDAMIDE, PSYCHOSIS CONNECTION

There's a reason CBD appears to improve psychosis in patients, and it all goes back to our old friend the endocannabinoid system (see page 30); in particular, the body's own cannabis-like chemical, anandamide.

We know that anandamide has an overall protective effect against stress and inflammation in the body, so scientists found it fascinating that in patients exhibiting psychosis for the first time, anandamide levels were eight times higher than control subjects.[99]

The first question they asked themselves was whether these skyrocketing anandamide levels were contributing to the psychosis itself. However, they soon realised there was an inverse relationship between anandamide levels and psychotic symptoms. So it seemed anandamide was just the body's way of trying to reverse psychosis.

Scientists had already observed how cannabis with high CBD content was associated with fewer psychotic episodes.[100] But could CBD be antipsychotic in itself?

A clinical study on 42 patients with schizophrenia gave them their answer. When CBD was administered, not only were the results comparable to the antipsychotic drug amisulpride, but patients experienced fewer unwanted side effects.[101] Interestingly, anandamide levels were elevated in the group given CBD, probably due to the inhibition of fatty acid amide hydrolase, the enzyme that breaks anandamide down in the body. Which would all seem to point towards a potentially therapeutic relationship between CBD and increased anandamide levels in patients with psychosis.

WHAT'S THE EVIDENCE?

It's a rare luxury in CBD research to talk in terms of multiple clinical trials, but when it comes to CBD for psychosis, a number of human studies have proved the compound to be both safe and effective.

Most recently, two randomised clinical studies have examined whether CBD used alongside an existing antipsychotic medication was more effective than the antipsychotic on its own. The first found that giving patients 1000mg of CBD daily resulted in improved psychotic symptoms, cognitive function and motor speed, compared to the control group who just received the antipsychotic.[102]

A similar study found no significant difference in psychosis symptoms or cognitive function when patients with chronic schizophrenia were given 600mg alongside their antipsychotic medication. However, CBD was found to be well tolerated.[103]

Unfortunately, no studies have progressed onto the third phase of clinical trials testing CBD as an antipsychotic drug on larger-sized groups of patients. Unless this happens and the positive results are replicated, CBD will not be considered an approved antipsychotic medication. So, watch this space!

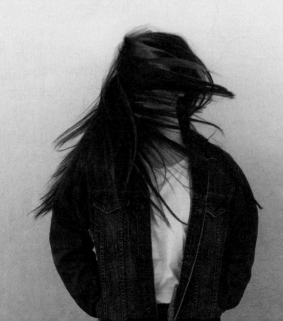

PTSD

There's very little good to be said about stress. When chronic, it can be a contributing factor to everything from heart disease to cancer. If it occurs after witnessing or experiencing a traumatic event as in PTSD, stress can lead to flashbacks, depression, anxiety, drug and alcohol misuse and sleep disorders.

The endocannabinoid system (ECS) is key to mitigating against the effects of stress. Indeed, in 1998, leading cannabinoid research scientist Professor Vincenzo Di Marzo describes how the ECS helps us 'relax, eat, sleep, forget and protect'.[104]

If we consider some of the symptoms of PTSD – the reliving of traumatic events, recurrent nightmares, depression and anxiety – one could imagine how something has gone awry with the endocannabinoid system's protective power.

In fact, one study measuring anandamide levels in subjects who were close to the World Trade Centre during the 9/11 attacks found those who had PTSD had lower anandamide levels than those who did not.[105]

We know that chronic stress tends to deplete the endocannabinoid system, limiting its ability to extinguish fearful memories from traumatic events. We also know that long-term stress causes an increase in fatty acid amide hydrolase (FAAH). Why does this matter? Well, FAAH breaks down anandamide in the body, so the more FAAH

is produced, the lower the circulating levels of anandamide, leaving us vulnerable to depression and anxiety.

It's proposed, then, that targeting the ECS could provide a new avenue for PTSD treatment going forward.[106]

CBD AND PTSD

While some PTSD sufferers have self-medicated with cannabis for many years, researchers believe that CBD-rich strains could be a safer, more effective way to ameliorate trauma symptoms.

Not least because CBD is a FAAH inhibitor. So, by introducing CBD into the body, less FAAH is produced, anandamide doesn't get broken down so quickly, allowing the 'feel good' endocannabinoid to do its mood-boosting, anxiety-reducing work for longer.

With the endocannabinoid system strengthened, it's hoped the ECS can get back to doing its important work of helping us relax, eat, sleep, forget and protect.

WHAT'S THE EVIDENCE?

While most of the early research into cannabis and PTSD focused on patients who were taking cannabis containing THC, one retrospective case series recorded the experiences of 11 adult patients with PTSD who were given CBD at an outpatient clinic.[107]

While some PTSD sufferers have self-medicated with cannabis for many years, researchers believe that CBD-rich strains could be a safer, more effective way to ameliorate trauma symptoms.

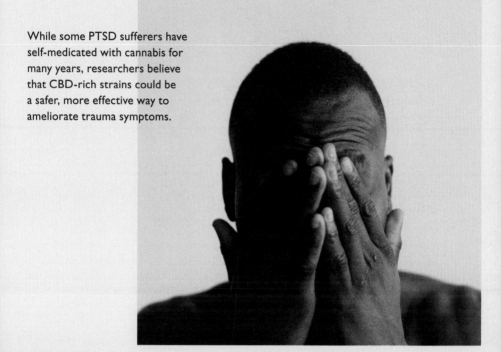

Encouragingly, 91 per cent of the patients experienced a reduction in symptom severity after 8 weeks of treatment with CBD. However, this was not a double-blind placebo study, and no precise dosing regime was established. But it was certainly enough to suggest CBD could be a well-tolerated and effective PTSD treatment of the future.

A new avenue of research also suggests that if given shortly after a traumatic event, CBD may reduce the likelihood of developing PTSD. Administering CBD to mice up to one hour after exposure to some kind of fearful event, was seen to prevent fear-based memories from consolidating.[108]

While this has yet to be studied in humans, it could mean taking CBD oil immediately after a traumatic event has occurred could limit the negative psychological impact.

SKIN CONDITIONS

Adding CBD to beauty products has been one of the hot trends of the last couple of years. While there's no evidence CBD is going to rid you of your wrinkles, the compound does show promise for bringing relief to some skin conditions such as psoriasis, eczema and acne.

WHY CBD?

Thanks to the presence of endocannabinoid receptors in our skin, we know that our ECS is involved in maintaining healthy skin-cell growth. When this becomes out of whack, it's thought skin conditions such as acne, excessively oily skin, allergic dermatitis, itchiness, psoriasis, hair growth disorders and even skin cancer can arise.

It's one reason CBD, with its ability to indirectly activate the endocannabinoid system, may have an overall therapeutic effect on many skin conditions.

Another key factor is that CBD has an overall anti-inflammatory effect. Many of us have experienced some kind of allergic reaction to a skincare product we've used (known as contact dermatitis), when an area of our skin becomes red and itchy. This is our immune system becoming activated.

In the case of psoriasis, the inflammation and itchiness is caused by an overactive immune system attacking its own tissues and not in response to any external allergen. Hence its classification as an autoimmune disease. The fact that CBD has an overall immunosuppressive effect means it could reduce the redness and itchiness associated with both conditions.[109] But that's not the end of CBD's benefits.

Preclinical studies show that CBD reduces excess oil production in skin, with researchers concluding the cannabinoid may well be a therapeutic agent for acne. CBD also has antibacterial properties, something of interest to anyone whose pimple has ever got infected, leading to scarring.[110]

WHAT'S THE EVIDENCE?

Conclusive clinical data doesn't exist right now showing CBD is effective for problem-skin issues. However, one small study following 20 patients with dermatitis and psoriasis applying CBD balm over 3 months, did throw up some encouraging results.[111]

All of the patients in the study had failed to find relief for their skin conditions using conventional treatments. However, all 20 saw improvements in skin elasticity and hydration, as well fewer lesions in the case of psoriasis, and less scarring in acne patients. Crucially, no allergic reactions or irritants were noted during the study.

If you are considering using a CBD cream or ointment for your skin condition, be sure to do a patch test beforehand.

STROKE AND BRAIN DAMAGE

Ask the average person on the street what they know about cannabis and the brain and most will say cannabis damages brain cells. In fact, for anyone over the age of 25, compounds in the plant can actually have the opposite effect.

That's because cannabinoids like CBD are considered neuroprotectants, meaning they actually protect our brains due to their antioxidant and anti-inflammatory properties.

When a stroke or head injury occurs, the brain is flooded by a type of neurotransmitter called glutamate. Excessive glutamate production causes excitotoxicity, a process by which brain cells are damaged and killed. So, scientists are on the lookout for ways to reduce glutamate production after strokes or head injuries, thereby limiting any brain damage that might occur.

And, it seems, CBD may fit the bill as it limits glutamate release by increasing anandamide signalling. CBD's activation of the 5-HT1A serotonin receptors also appears to have a neuroprotective effect, which researchers believe may lead to improvement in cognitive and functional impairment after strokes and brain injuries.[112]

WHAT'S THE EVIDENCE?

Strokes

Strokes occur when a thickening of the arteries prevents enough blood from reaching the brain. The resulting damage, known as ischemic injury, can include brain cell death, partial paralysis and loss of speech.

So far, research into whether CBD can limit brain damage caused after a stroke has only reached preclinical stage. Results, however, have been promising, with CBD administration improving long-term functional recovery, reducing neuronal loss and modulating cell death, excitotoxicity and neuro-inflammation in a rat model of ischemic arterial stroke.[113]

Traumatic Brain Injury

Traumatic Brain Injury (TBI) is a debilitating condition caused by a severe blow to the head. Aside from the initial effects such as severe concussion, symptoms can be more long-lasting and include cognitive and behavioural issues, mobility difficulties, problems with speech, visual impairment, painful headaches and drastic mood changes.

Right now, there are more anecdotal accounts about CBD's efficacy in improving recovery after TBI than scientific studies. However, it's thought the same neuroprotective principles apply.

In the United States, a study is currently recruiting to see whether a hemp-based CBD oil improves wellbeing, sleep quality, cognitive ability and changes in neuronal activity or stress biomarkers after TBI. But it will be a long time before any results are published.[114]

Chronic Traumatic Encephalopathy

Chronic traumatic encephalopathy (CTE), an incurable degenerative brain disease caused by repeated trauma such as concussions, is linked to sports such as rugby, football, boxing and American football.

With inflammation in the brain being a common marker in CTE, it's not surprising that CBD's anti-inflammatory and brain-protective effects make it a potential palliative treatment.

CTE is a particular problem among professional NFL players. One survey found 9 in 10 former players had concussion while playing football and two-thirds of those said they experience continuing symptoms.[115] While not a CTE sufferer himself, ex-Baltimore Ravens player Eugene Monroe has donated $80,000 to CBD research, with a particular focus on the use of CBD to alleviate the symptoms of CTE.

Neonatal Hypoxic-Ischemic Encephalopathy (Infant Brain Damage)

One of the most extensively investigated areas of research into CBD and brain damage actually involves giving the cannabis compound to newborn infants.

You're probably thinking, 'how can it be OK to give CBD to babies?' CBD,

given alongside the current treatment, hypothermia (reducing the baby's body temperature to 33–34°C), might just save the lives of hundreds of thousands of babies who die each year due to oxygen starvation during or after birth.

After preclinical studies on piglets showed combining CBD and hypothermia increased infant survival from 60 per cent to nearly 100 per cent, Spanish researchers recently got the go-ahead to start a clinical trial in the UK and Spain.[116]

Purified CBD will be given to newborn babies intravenously alongside hypothermia as soon as infant brain damage is detected. CBD may extend the therapeutic window (which is only six hours after birth for hypothermia) as the cannabinoid has been found to be neuroprotective when administered for up to 24 hours after brain injury occurred in newborn mice.[117]

Despite promising evidence for CBD's neuroprotective effects, administering CBD oil after any form of brain injury should not be considered without a prior discussion with your doctor.

04

CBD FOR WELLNESS

The Western world is mad about wellness, with the industry worth $4.5 trillion globally. Over the past 50 years, we've left mere survival behind and are now concerned with how to be the best, most successful versions of ourselves.

However, with economic advancement invariably comes high levels of stress. It's as if all that striving has left us burned out and in need of some nurturing care. Something provided by the wellness industry – from offerings based on ancient traditions such as yoga, mindfulness and fasting, to the more faddish colonics, cow hugging and activated charcoal. So how does CBD fit into all this?

Right now, according to the Centre for Medical Cannabis, approximately 6.5 million people in the UK have tried CBD.[118] If we consider that about half the UK population don't take any prescription medication, it's possible to extrapolate that around 3 million people are using CBD for wellness purposes.

But what does it mean to take CBD for wellness?

Marketing plays a massive role in the wellness industry, with companies paying for their products to be associated with social-media influencers and celebrities. So inevitably, when it comes to CBD, there will be a proportion who use CBD oil because it's cool. However, the majority of us probably take CBD to help us cope with the stress of modern life; to feel a little calmer, sleep better; and as a natural alternative for any minor aches and pains we suffer.

So, let's take a look at how CBD can enhance our overall wellbeing and quality of life by improving our mood, helping us cope better with stress, feeling more focused and even doing a better workout at the gym.

CBD FOR STRESS

MANAGEMENT

We are in the midst of a stress epidemic. One mental health survey found 74 per cent of the UK felt overwhelmed or unable to cope in the last year,[119] while stress causes around one million Americans to miss work every day.[120]

Stress feels bad enough in itself, but the fact that it can cause a number of health conditions such as heart disease, cancer, depression and anxiety, gastrointestinal problems and diabetes, means it's vital to find effective ways to manage our own stress levels.

But life is inherently stressful. Society has programmed us to strive to have it all: the perfect job, the perfect family, the perfect house. Only there is no 'perfect'. It's something constructed to keep us working more. Then throw in life's inevitable curveballs, such as the death of a loved one, or our own serious illness, and it's no wonder we're all on the point of physical and mental collapse.

THE ENDOCANNABINOID SYSTEM AND STRESS

The endocannabinoid system (ECS) plays a key role in protecting us against stress.[121] Indeed, endocannabinoid signalling is found throughout areas related to stress, in particular

the hypothalamic-pituitary-adrenal (HPA) axis, which is responsible for controlling cortisol and other stress hormones. Endocannabinoid receptors have also been discovered in the amygdala, part of the limbic system of the brain involved in processing emotions and memory, particularly fear.

When our ECS successfully modulates the HPA axis and amygdala, it allows the body to cope with high stress levels, while disrupted ECS signalling can lead to an inability to adapt to chronic stress, making us more vulnerable to depression.

Interestingly, prolonged exposure to stress can cause a reduction in anandamide levels (the 'bliss' endocannabinoid) and a downregulation in the CB1 endocannabinoid receptor. CBD is thought to strengthen endocannabinoid tone by increasing anandamide signalling, giving our ECS a helping hand in mitigating against the negative effects of stress in the body.

CBD MAY PROTECT US AGAINST STRESS

Encouragingly, it also seems that CBD can have a more direct effect on stress by increasing serotonin signalling in our brain, causing us to feel less anxious. Plus, by calming our sympathetic nervous system, CBD may have the knock-on effect of protecting us against stress-related heart disease.

An overactivated amygdala can result in artery inflammation, and a higher risk of heart attack.[122] With repeated stress, our bone marrow produces extra white blood cells, which in turn triggers inflammation and the build-up of artery-clogging plaque. So the fact that CBD is anti-inflammatory could also be good for the health of our stressed-out hearts. CBD's ability to calm our nervous system may also explain why initial studies suggest it limits increases in blood pressure occurring in stressful situations.[123]

Anecdotally, CBD users report feeling less overwhelmed, more able to cope, and a greater sense of overall calm. So, it's possible, then, for anyone going through a period of intense stress, that CBD could provide buffer against the most immediate and unpleasant effects, as well as protecting the body from any harmful long-term damage caused by stress.

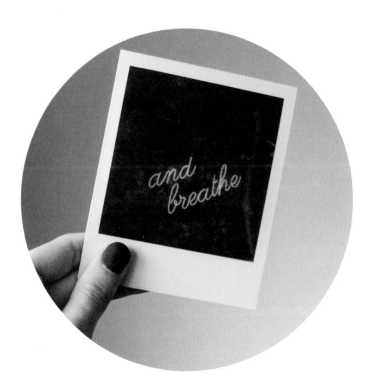

THE CBD BOOK

CBD FOR SLEEP

Sleep disorders such as insomnia affect between 50 and 70 million adults in the United States[124] and, when chronic, increase the risk of heart disease, obesity and diabetes. Plus there's the knock-on effect to mental health with higher associated rates of depression and anxiety.

Stress is a major contributing factor. Unfortunately, it can all become a rather vicious circle. After several days of restricted sleep, levels of the stress hormone cortisol shoot up in the early evening – just at the time when they are normally dropping in preparation for a sound night's sleep.[125]

Many people report experiencing better sleep when taking CBD, although there is limited data proving CBD an effective treatment for sleep disorders. One large retrospective study did find that most of the 72 patients with both anxiety and poor sleep benefited from taking CBD, although the improvements in anxiety were better sustained over time.[126]

Again CBD's impact on stress and anxiety through the activation of the 5-HTP1 serotonin receptors may well help people sleep better. If we're feeling less anxious, there's less chance of us waking up at 4am in a cold sweat. And remember the stress hormone cortisol? CBD has also been found to interfere with cortisol secretion, causing sensations of sedation.[127] CBD is known to have a biphasic effect.

In the context of sleep, this tends to mean that at low doses CBD can cause alertness, while at higher doses, people feel sleepy.

So if you are trying CBD for the first time to aid sleep, leave a couple of hours before hitting the sack to see how you react. It's also worth noting that certain terpenes like limonene can have an uplifting effect, so if you're using CBD oil for sleep, try to find an oil light on limonene and containing more myrcene (the terpene that gives the 'couch lock' effect in marijuana).

'In the context of sleep, this tends to mean that at low doses CBD can cause alertness, while at higher doses, people feel sleepy.'

CBD AND WOMEN'S HEALTH

According to the Project CBD 'Cultivating Wellness Survey', there is a certain amount of gender bias surrounding CBD with 62.4 per cent of responders being women,[128] a result mirrored in a similar survey carried out by the Brightfield Group.[129] That's not to say that taking health supplements is a wholly female lifestyle choice. Statistically, roughly the same proportion of men and women take dietary supplements (77 per cent of women and 73 per cent of men).[130]

This female skew may reflect the fact that the two most commonly stated reasons for using CBD – pain and anxiety – affect women disproportionately. Plus, they are also commonly experienced with issues concerning women's hormonal and reproductive health, such as endometriosis, premenstrual syndrome, period pain and the menopause.

Many women report that using CBD during the menopause helps them weather the choppy waters this stage in life brings to their emotional landscape. Indeed, celebrity menopause and lifestyle guru Meg Matthews found CBD so effective at managing her hormone-driven anxiety and insomnia, she started her own CBD brand.

A number of women-focused CBD products have sprung up on the market, offering CBD suppositories (inserted vaginally or anally) and even CBD tampons

to bring relief to the discomfort experienced during menstruation.

While scientific evidence remains scant proving CBD balances women's hormones, the fact that it helps support our endocannabinoid system, which regulates all biological activity including our hormones, may mean that taking CBD could be a way to smooth the jagged edges of our sometimes hormonally challenged internal world.

'Many women report that using CBD during the menopause helps them weather the choppy waters this stage in life brings to their emotional landscape.'

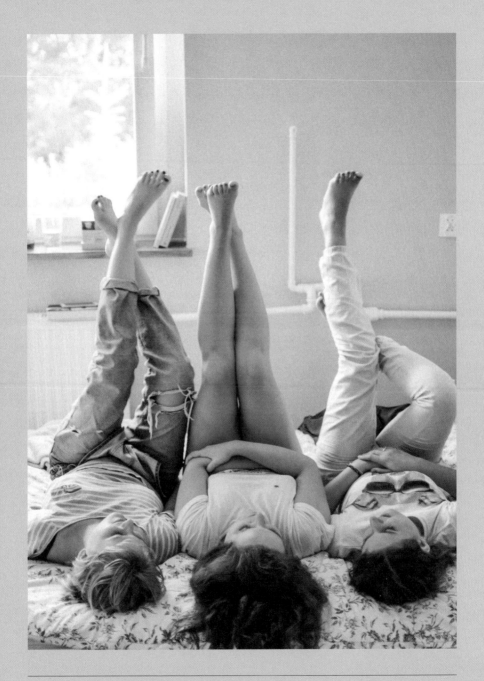

CBD FOR FOCUS AND
CONCENTRATION

Many people believe CBD can be used to aid focus.

Of late, the CBD wellness trend has been hitting the world of superstar DJs. Over the years, many of them have been around the block a bit, gathering a few vices along the way, but are now living the dream of a clean lifestyle.

Only DJing in clubs at 4am isn't exactly conducive to keeping on the straight and narrow. Interestingly a select few have replaced their rum and coke (insert here any other recreational drug of choice) with CBD oil saying it gives them better focus.

That's because CBD is increasingly considered a nootropic – a 'smart drug' that improves cognitive function, concentration, memory, creativity or motivation in healthy subjects. It's a reason why CBD oil is the hot new ingredient in 'functional' foods and drinks designed to maximise brain power. Although right now, there's no scientific evidence to back up the biohacking marketing claims.

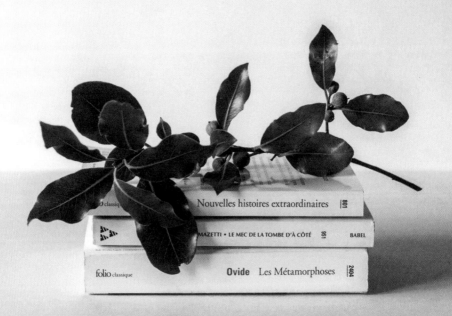

Nouvelles histoires extraordinaires

MAZETTI • LE MEC DE LA TOMBE D'À CÔTÉ   BABEL

folio classique   **Ovide** Les Métamorphoses

CBD AS A SPORTS
SUPPLEMENT

Playing sports and going to the gym are key pillars of the wellness industry. But did you know many gym goers and athletes are incorporating CBD into their training routine?

It shouldn't be a surprise when you consider the relationship between high-impact physical exercise and the endocannabinoid system. Scientists have measured notable increases in the bliss endocannabinoid anandamide after sustained cardiovascular exercise, totally turning on its head the perceived wisdom that endorphins are responsible for the euphoria experienced through exercise.[131]

Over in the United States, NFL football players have been singing CBD's praises for a while, saying the compound helps them recover better from injury, and it is particularly prevalent among mixed martial arts competitors, many of whom are sponsored by CBD companies.

CBD BEFORE AND AFTER A WORKOUT

Let's face it: for many of us, just getting to the gym is a miracle in itself, so once we're there we want to make the most of our workout. How does CBD fit into this?

Scientific data is pretty sparse proving whether CBD does actually make us train better. However, the overwhelming consensus from anecdotal accounts is that CBD improves concentration, focus and stamina – all key components of an effective workout.

CBD is also finding favour among the bodybuilding community, as it may promote the creation of muscle mass, or at least limit the breaking down of muscle caused by the stress hormone cortisol.

Because CBD is analgesic and anti-inflammatory, it could also give that extra boost to a workout by allowing athletes to push through the pain barrier.

And what about CBD and recovery? Top international rugby player Dom Day became a CBD convert after it helped him recover from knee surgery. So much so that he went on to set up his own CBD company with his friend and fellow Saracens player, George Kruis.

CBD AND BEAUTY

We know that CBD has a therapeutic effect on skin conditions such as psoriasis and acne, which is thanks to its anti-inflammatory and antioxidant properties. So, it was only a matter of time before CBD made the jump to the non-medical skincare world, where fighting off free radicals and calming irritated skin are the holy grails of the anti-ageing business.

Ignoring the question of whether beauty products themselves are little more than marketing smoke and mirrors, does adding CBD make them any more effective?

My sense is that including CBD in the list of ingredients is an excuse to hop on the CBD billion-dollar bandwagon, as there's certainly no evidence to suggest CBD has any anti-ageing properties. And don't get me started on the likes of CBD beard oil and CBD shampoo. More fool you if you get sucked in.

That said, one recent report suggested that by 2024, CBD skincare is likely to represent 10 per cent of the global skincare market.[132] So it looks like in the not-too-distant future we'll all be slathering our faces in CBD facemasks.

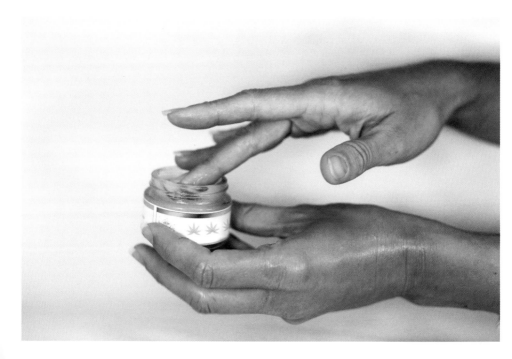

05

HOW TO
TAKE CBD

Whether taking CBD oil for wellness reasons or to help manage symptoms of a health condition, we're all left with the same questions:

— How do I find the right CBD product for me?
— How much CBD should I take?
— Will CBD interact with my prescription medication?
— Is CBD safe to take long term?

In this chapter, I'll explain all the confusing terminology like 'full spectrum', 'CBD isolate' and 'terpenes'; I'll go through the different delivery methods such as tinctures, capsules and vaping; and give you an easy step-by-step guide on how to find the best CBD product for you.

You'll also get tips on finding the correct CBD dosage for you, maximising CBD absorption in the body and what to expect when you take CBD for the first time.

This is perhaps the most practical section of the book, empowering you to feel fully equipped so that you can confidently begin your own CBD journey.

CHOOSING A CBD PRODUCT

You've decided that CBD might just be for you and have typed into Google 'buy CBD'. To your horror 822,000,000 results come back from thousands of CBD companies all shouting loudest about why their products are the best.

Not only that, you come across terms like 'full spectrum', 'whole plant' and 'CBD isolate'. They're bandied about with such ease, as if everyone knows perfectly well what they mean. Only you don't. You just want to buy CBD oil.

So what's the difference?

You're probably thinking, if CBD is so great, I'll just buy the strongest, purest CBD I can find. However, in the CBD world, things don't work that way. In fact, it's best to think of CBD oil's benefits as coming from the sum of all its parts. That's why most CBD oils on the market are 'full-spectrum' or 'whole-plant' CBD oils, containing not only cannabidiol, but a host of minor cannabinoids (including THC), terpenes and flavonoids.

Increasingly, though, companies are also offering 'zero THC' CBD products called 'broad spectrum' CBD oils, while a minority use purified CBD, also known as 'CBD isolate', in their products.

FULL-SPECTRUM CBD OIL

Current wisdom suggests that taking CBD extracts where the natural balance of cannabinoids, terpenes and flavonoids found in cannabis has been preserved, offers the most benefits to our health.

In order to do this, the extraction process has to be carefully managed in order to ensure that key ingredients are not lost.

Most CBD oils on the market have been extracted using some kind of solvent, either high pressure CO^2 or ethanol, which act to separate the hemp trichomes (where the cannabinoids are made) from the plant material.

The dark, sticky hemp extract known as 'CBD crude' is then filtered during a process called winterisation, in which any plant waxes or chlorophyll is removed. Next, comes decarboxylation where gentle heat turns CBDA (CBD's acidic precursor) into CBD, all the while carefully avoiding any unnecessary damage to unstable molecules such as the aromatic terpenes.

The resulting extract is rich in CBD, but also contains other key compounds, such as the cannabinoids cannabigerol (CBG), cannabidivarin (CBDV), cannabichromene (CBC) and legally allowed amounts of tetrahydrocannabinol (THC). Some CBD oils also contain acidic cannabinoids that have not been through the heat process, such as CBDA and THCA.

But the full-spectrum CBD oil story doesn't end there. Terpenes, the molecules responsible for the fragrance in aromatic plants, also play a key role.

Many of us will have experienced the relaxing effects of lavender oil or felt uplifted after breathing in the invigorating aroma of lemons and oranges.

These physiological effects are caused by terpenes like linalool in lavender and limonene in citrus fruit, both of which can be found in the hemp plant, alongside other terpenes such as pinene, myrcene and beta caryophyllene.

BROAD-SPECTRUM CBD OIL

Many people feel uncomfortable taking CBD oil containing THC. Perhaps they're worried about failing a drugs test or they just don't like the idea of taking an intoxicating substance, even if it's just in trace amounts.

Considering the number of times CBD oils have been tested to contain over the legal 0.2 per cent (0.3 per cent in the US) of THC, it's understandable consumers have been crying out for a zero THC CBD oil. So with the arrival of broad-spectrum CBD oil on the market, it seems like their prayers have been answered.

Many companies market their broad-spectrum products as the same as full spectrum, just without the THC. Full-spectrum purists disagree, however, insisting the trace levels of THC in true full-spectrum oils are required to benefit from the much-celebrated 'entourage effect' (see page 88).

There are two types of broad-spectrum products:

1. 'True' broad-spectrum products where THC has been removed using chromatography or distillation, leaving the other compounds intact.

2. Fake' broad-spectrum products using CBD isolate but adding in cannabinoids and terpenes afterwards.

Unfortunately, for consumers it is almost impossible to differentiate between the two, short of contacting the CBD company directly and asking them outright. Even then there's no guarantee they themselves will know and can give you a straight answer.

CBD ISOLATE

Which brings me nicely onto CBD isolate. CBD isolate is a crystalline white powder that has had all the other naturally occurring molecules in hemp removed. So it's literally CBD and nothing else.

Cheap CBD isolate from India and China has flooded the market recently, and is an attractive option for anyone wanting to make a quick buck in the CBD-oil 'green rush'. CBD isolate is also commonly used in CBD skincare and beauty products because it is water soluble.

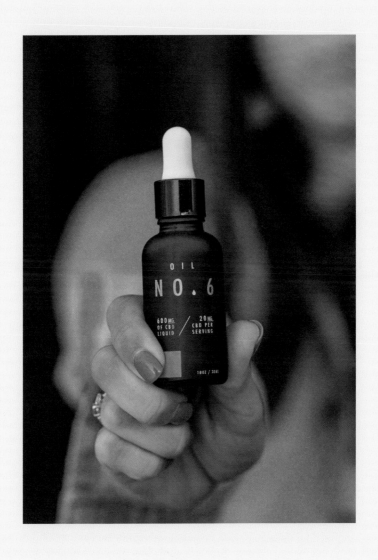

If you've read the CBD research section earlier in the book, you'll have seen that most studies use relatively high doses of CBD isolate, otherwise known as purified CBD. It's therefore understandable to assume as a CBD consumer that you should choose a CBD isolate product in order to get the best results.

However, counterintuitively, CBD users report experiencing less beneficial effects from CBD isolate products or require higher CBD doses in order to get the same results as a full-spectrum CBD oil.

The Entourage Effect – Fact or Fiction?
If you speak to a researcher involved in drug development, they will probably say that the benefits enjoyed by CBD consumers around the world are due to the placebo effect – whereby any positive effects are caused by the belief that CBD will make them feel better rather than the CBD itself.

From a pharmacological perspective, CBD's lack of potency at its biological targets means far higher concentrations than those taken by CBD oil consumers are needed to get any physiological effects.

And yet, huge numbers of people do indeed find relief for symptoms as varied as pain, anxiety, autoimmune conditions, autism and epilepsy with as little as 10mg of CBD a day.

How could this be?

Current thinking suggests a synergy between all the compounds in the cannabis plant – known as the entourage effect – may be the answer.

Interestingly, the term 'entourage effect' first came into being to describe how seemingly inactive metabolites in the endocannabinoid system increase the activity of the endocannabinoids anandamide and 2-AG.[133]

The concept was later extended to the cannabis plant by Dr Ethan Russo in his paper, 'Taming THC: potential cannabis synergy and phytocannabinoid-terpenoid entourage effects.'[134] He proposed a unique 'herbal synergy' between the minor cannabinoids, terpenes and flavonoids, which act to potentiate the effects of the cannabis plant's protagonists, THC and CBD.

This was music to the ears of the artisan cannabis oil community. Suddenly there was a respected scientist saying that whole-plant cannabis is the most effective form and not the single cannabinoids commonly used in scientific research.

That said, outright proof showing the theory's validity is currently lacking. One meta-analysis comparing full-spectrum CBD-rich extracts and purified CBD in refractory epilepsy found full-spectrum CBD products more effective.[135] Patients taking the CBD-rich extracts had better seizure control, required a lower dosage and experienced fewer side effects than those using purified CBD.

Another preclinical study comparing the anti-tumoral effects of purified THC and a full-spectrum cannabis extract containing THC in breast cancer cell lines, showed the botanical cannabis extract to have superior anti-cancer effects.[136]

Certainly on the whole, full-spectrum CBD oils continue to be more popular amongst CBD consumers. One would assume that if the cheaper CBD isolate-based products were comparable, this full-spectrum market would have dried up by now.

Anecdotal accounts appear to back up the entourage effect, with some CBD consumers actively seeking out the 'lesser ingredients' like certain minor cannabinoids or terpenes in their CBD oil of choice because they say they make them more effective.

For most of us, though, our knowledge doesn't reach that far. We just want to make sure the product we buy contains the amount of CBD it says on the label and is free from any hidden nasties like pesticides, heavy metals or mould.

Look for a Certificate of Analysis
CBD oils have had a bit of bad press recently. A number of reports testing the content of over-the-counter CBD oils have found a few brands contained less CBD oil than advertised, and in one case, a CBD product sold in a high-street pharmacy contained no CBD oil at all.[137]

Because UK law does not allow domestic hemp farmers to use or sell hemp flowers – the parts of the plant containing all the cannabinoid good stuff – most CBD oil on sale has been imported from producers or suppliers in the EU or the US.

A lot of processes have already happened by the time this CBD oil reaches the UK: harvesting, extraction, winterisation, decarboxylation and distillation. Getting a final product containing just the right amount of CBD, legally allowed amounts of THC, plus all the other minor cannabinoids and terpenes present in a full-spectrum oil requires expertise, scientific rigour and some extremely expensive machinery. And in the wild, wild west that is the CBD industry, precise cannabinoid content is not necessarily guaranteed.

'Current wisdom suggests that taking CBD extracts where the natural balance of cannabinoids, terpenes and flavonoids found in cannabis has been preserved offers the most benefits to our health.'

So any CBD company worth its salt will only source CBD products that come with a certificate of analysis (COA) clearly showing the cannabinoid (and ideally terpene) profile, as well as contaminant testing proving they are free from heavy metals, herbicides, pesticides and fungicides, bacteria or fungus.

Unfortunately, due to the unregulated nature of the CBD industry, inconsistencies in results are commonplace from different laboratories testing the same products. So, opting for a government-accredited laboratory is perhaps the best way to guarantee accuracy.[138]

Many CBD companies pay for their own third-party lab reports, and links to COAs can often be found on their websites. However, it should be noted that not all COAs are created equal and 'fudging' can occur.

If you decide to check out a COA before buying your CBD oil, here are a few points to consider:

1. Does the COA come from a government-accredited lab? If not, is the lab EN ISO/IEC 17025 compliant (the internationally recognised gold-standard that shows a lab to be technically competent)?

2. Does the COA come from an independent third-party lab (and not in-house)?

3. Check the date – if it's from two years ago, the COA probably doesn't correspond to the CBD batch your product comes from (or if it does correspond, perhaps wonder why the company isn't selling much product).

4. Check that the COA has been issued to the company you are buying your CBD oil from, and if not, that it's for the supplier they sourced their CBD oil from.

5. Has any information on the COA been blacked out? If so, warning bells should sound about the validity of the certificate.

In an attempt to make the CBD market more transparent, some states in the US require CBD companies to provide QR codes on their product labels, which when scanned by an app on a smartphone, link to COAs, product ingredients, quality-control methods and expiry dates. A few UK CBD companies are also beginning to include QR codes on labelling, and in a future regulated CBD market, QR codes may be on all UK CBD products.

In the meantime, checking a COA is an important part of your research prior to choosing a CBD product. So don't be afraid to ask a company if there's nothing obvious on their website directing you to a COA for your particular CBD oil product. If they can't provide you with the documentation, it may well be a sign they're actually not 'the number one trusted CBD provider' they say they are.

GETTING MAXIMUM BANG FOR YOUR BUCK – WHY BIOAVAILABILITY MATTERS

Choosing a CBD product is a mind-boggling process with an infinite number of CBD products, flavours and strengths on the market. Understanding the term 'bioavailability' – how much CBD is used by the body – is key to making an informed decision about which CBD product is best for you.

Bioavailability is defined as 'the proportion of a substance that enters the bloodstream when introduced into the body and so is able to have an active effect'.

Indeed, it's imperative to know the bioavailability of a drug in order to determine standard dosage. Take, for instance, paracetamol which has a bioavailability of between 60 and 70 per cent. This means 60 to 70 per cent of the paracetamol taken orally by patients reaches the bloodstream and can be used by the body.

Because CBD is non-water soluble, it has quite low bioavailability, on average somewhere between 10 and 20 per cent. Our bodies are approximately 60 per cent water and, as we all know, oil and water do not mix. So in most cases, more than 80 per cent of the CBD oil you take never makes it into your bloodstream and is essentially wasted.

Why does this matter? CBD oil can be expensive, with a 10ml bottle of low-strength (300mg) CBD oil costing around £25 and a higher strength oil (1500mg) a whopping £120. So maximising bioavailability is a way of getting the most bang for your buck. By increasing the amount of CBD your body can use, you essentially don't need to take as much product and can therefore spend less of your hard-earned cash. But how can we increase CBD bioavailability?

Choosing a water-soluble CBD product is one way, with CBD companies claiming an increase in bioavailability of up to five times compared to standard CBD oil. Water-soluble CBD is created by breaking CBD molecules down into nano-sized particles, so they're easily dissolved in water. That said, the majority of CBD products on the market are still non-water soluble. So what else can we do?

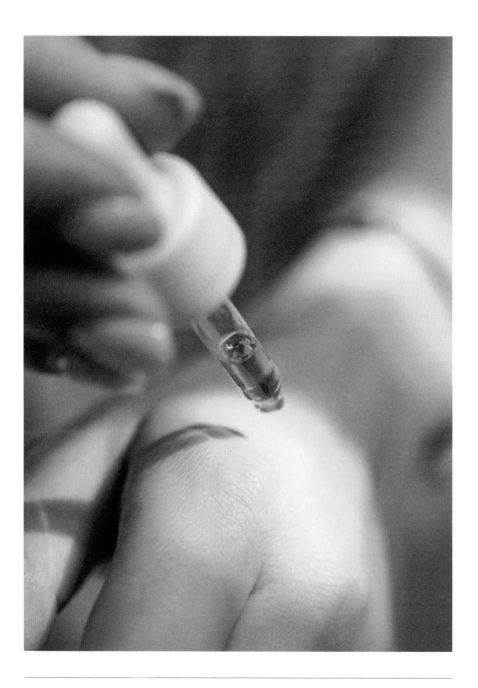

THE CBD BOOK

BEST DELIVERY METHODS FOR CBD BIOAVAILABILITY

The way we take CBD, also known as the delivery method, can also increase bioavailability. So whether you choose to take CBD in capsules, under the tongue as an oil or vape it straight into the lungs affects how much CBD your body absorbs.

In basic terms, the fewer steps there are between ingesting CBD and the compound entering the bloodstream, the higher the absorption rate.

1. Vaping CBD
Since the CBD passes directly into the lungs, this method has the highest bioavailability: somewhere between 30 and 50 per cent.

2. CBD drops taken sublingually
CBD oil or tinctures taken under the tongue are absorbed by highly permeable salivary glands that are rich in blood supply. This method offers absorption rates of between 12 to 35 per cent.

3. CBD taken orally (capsules, edibles)
Taking CBD in capsules or in edibles has the lowest bioavailability, with absorption rates of between 4 to 20 per cent. On swallowing, CBD has to pass through the digestive system, where much of the CBD is broken down by liver enzymes.

4. Topical or Transdermal CBD
Calculating the bioavailability of CBD is far from being an exact science, and little data exists about applying CBD to the skin. In theory, it should be difficult for a bog-standard CBD oil to penetrate the skin's layers and reach joints or muscles below. And yet, many people with arthritis report finding benefit from rubbing CBD oils and balms into their painful joints. New CBD formulations that penetrate the skin are being developed to be used in patches and in gels.

'The fewer steps there are between ingesting CBD and the compound entering the bloodstream, the higher the absorption rate.'

WHAT TYPES OF CBD

PRODUCT ARE AVAILABLE?

One of the questions I am most frequently asked is which type of CBD product should I buy?

On the whole, we're used to taking our medication and health supplements in capsule form, so anything that comes in drops or you have to inhale feels immediately alien.

But it's important to remember that only 70 years or so ago, before the pharmaceutical industry took hold, doctors regularly prescribed herbal medicine to their patients in tincture form.

To this day, if you're a fan of herbal medicines like St John's wort, echinacea or ginkgo biloba, they are usually available in capsule or tincture form. Most of us probably choose the capsules for convenience. But for better absorption and more flexibility in dosing, we should always go for a tincture. Only, no one in the average health food store actually tells us that.

So perhaps when we're taking CBD oil, we should treat it in the same way as an herbal medicine – a bit harsh on the palate, but worth taking in its most natural, unadulterated form.

CBD OIL DROPS AND TINCTURES

OK, to kick off, let's just clarify the difference between CBD oil drops and tinctures. CBD tinctures are made by suspending hemp flowers in distilled alcohol, and are usually mixed with glycerine, as well as flavourings to make them more palatable.

In reality, most of the CBD oil available in the UK has been extracted using high pressure CO_2 or ethanol as a solvent. The thick hemp extract is then winterised (filtered to remove any plant waxes and chlorophyll), decarboxylated, and then mixed with a carrier oil such as hemp seed oil, MCT oil or olive oil. However, CBD oil and CBD tinctures are both administered in the same way: using a dropper under the tongue.

Advantages

CBD oil taken sublingually has good absorption rates. It also offers more flexibility when it comes to dosing, as it allows you to increase your dose by one milligram at a time, although this is only possible with a low-strength oil.

Disadvantages

If you're not a fan of the very distinctive hemp taste, CBD drops can seem unpalatable. Sometimes CBD oil bottles can leak – not so great if you carry one in your pocket or handbag.

Instructions for Use

Stand in front of a mirror (that way you can see when a drop lands under your tongue) and drop the CBD oil, drop by drop, under your tongue. Hold for one minute to ensure as much of the CBD as possible gets absorbed into the bloodstream. Try not to drink any liquids immediately afterwards.

Top Tip

Many CBD oils categorise their products in terms of CBD percentage of CBD. While that's nice to know, it's not helpful if you want an accurate dosage. So look for CBD brands that tell you not only how many milligrams of CBD there are in the bottle but also how much CBD is in each drop. To give an example, in a 10ml bottle containing 300mg of CBD, each drop will contain roughly 1mg of CBD. This is important if you're just starting out on your CBD journey, as following the 'start low and go slow' approach is impossible otherwise.

CBD CAPSULES OR SOFTGELS

Softgels are the go-to choice for anyone who struggles with the hempy taste of CBD oil drops or just wants the convenience of popping a pill in their mouth.

Advantages

CBD capsules are perhaps the most discreet and convenient way to take CBD. No hempy taste makes them easier on the palate. Plus you always know how much CBD you're taking, avoiding any 'was that one drop or two' mishaps often experienced with CBD oil drops.

Disadvantages

Inferior absorption rates put many more seasoned CBD pros off taking capsules, as does the length of time for them to take effect. The fixed dose can be advantageous, but doesn't allow for much flexibility when increasing your dose to find your 'sweet spot' (more on this later).

Instructions for Use

Take with or after food to increase bioavailability.

Top Tip

If you're intent on buying CBD capsules, opt for ones containing water-soluble CBD which can be absorbed by the body before reaching the stomach.

VAPING CBD

Vaping CBD is both popular and controversial at the same time. On the one hand, it has the fastest-acting effect and the best bioavailability, while on the other, vaping's safety has been called into question after over a thousand cases of vaping-related illnesses were reported in the United States.

When you vape CBD, a small heating element heats the CBD vape liquid, producing vapour,which is inhaled into the lungs through a mouthpiece.

There are essentially two kinds of vape devices: the tank style and vape pens.

Tank-style CBD vapes comprise a battery-heated disposable cartridge or a refillable container filled with CBD e-liquid. CBD is typically mixed with propylene glycol (PG) and vegetable glycerin (VG) to make it 'vapeable'. Terpenes or food-grade fruit flavourings may be added to enhance the vape experience. While some CBD e-liquids contain full-spectrum CBD, when it comes to vaping, CBD isolate may be the safer option as there is no risk of inhaling oil droplets – which is what has been linked to lipid pneumonia.

Those new to vaping tend to opt for preloaded vape pens, which as the name suggests, are the size and shape of a pen. Vape pens contain a battery, atomiser and are pre-loaded with cannabidiol-containing e-juice or CBD concentrate.

Is Vaping CBD Safe?

Again the lack of regulation in the CBD market means food-grade ingredients like MCT oil or vitamin E acetate have been added to CBD to make vape juice (another word for e-liquid). These are fine when swallowed, but not suitable for inhalation into our lungs. It is suspected their use may account for some of the vaping lung damage in the United States. Some controversy also surrounds PG and VG, which alongside the flavourings added to CBD vape juice, may also irritate the lungs. Vaping devices themselves are not without their own health concerns. A recent study found heavy metal by-products such as aluminium, calcium, chromium, copper, iron, lead, magnesium, nickel, silicon, tin and zinc in the vapour produced by high-voltage tank-style vapes. Furthermore, concentrations of certain metals, such as lead, increased with the higher voltage of the device.[139]

Questions of safety also surround the use of vape pens. Over time, the heating coil can slowly break down and oxidise, allowing metal nanoparticles to make it into the inhaled vapour.

Advantages

Vaping CBD is the fastest-acting delivery method and boasts the highest bioavailability. CBD is easily added to e-cigarette cartridges, making it a convenient and socially acceptable way to take CBD.

Disadvantages

Right now, the jury is out about vaping's safety profile. CBD is too often mixed with artificial ingredients and flavourings to make CBD e-liquid. Why mess with what nature has given us?

Instructions for Use

CBD e-liquid: shake well before each use. Read the instructions on how to fill the tank or cartridge. Inhale from the vaporiser and complete the breath. Hold for 10–20 seconds.

Top Tip

Vaping fancy flavours sounds fun, but make sure anything added into the vape liquid is as natural as possible and safe to inhale into your lungs. Only buy from companies that provide independent lab tests.

CBD SUPPOSITORIES

From one orifice to another: CBD suppositories are perhaps one of the less-frequently-used delivery methods for taking CBD.

Very few companies offer them and frankly most of us are not very comfortable putting 'food supplements' as a suppository. Indeed, there is some dispute over whether CBD suppositories could even be classed as a food supplement at all due to the hole/holes through which they are administered.

But if you are having trouble swallowing CBD oil for some reason, suppositories provide a useful alternative route of entry.

To make suppositories, CBD oil or extract is mixed with a medium, such as coconut oil, and encased in bullet-shaped plastic moulding. For easy insertion (rectal or vaginal), suppositories need to be refrigerated for the coconut oil to harden.

Advantages

Suppositories are reported to have superior bioavailability, with a reasonable proportion of CBD reaching the bloodstream within half an hour, although it remains unclear whether they only offer anything more than 'localised' relief. As mentioned previously, if keeping CBD oil down when taken orally is a problem, CBD suppositories are a good alternative.

Disadvantages

Most CBD suppositories are between 25 and 100mg, so using them to up-titrate (slowly increase your dose) isn't practical. Obviously, they aren't the most convenient delivery method and as a result tend to be used by those taking CBD medically.

Instructions for Use

Lie on your side with your bottom leg outstretched and the other leg bent and pulled towards your chest. Using protective gloves and lube if necessary, insert the suppository into the anal (or vaginal) passage, pushing past the sphincter muscle.

Top Tip

Suppositories are best used at night, as lying horizontally tends to help their absorption (whereas the downward pull of gravity doesn't).

CBD TOPICALS

CBD creams, balms and massage oils are an increasingly popular way of enjoying CBD's benefits. Many companies add extra natural ingredients, such as arnica and essential oils to bring relief to tired and aching muscles or calm irritated and inflamed skin.

Anecdotal reports abound, recounting so-and-so's elderly aunt who after rubbing her arthritic joints with CBD cream, started knitting again for the first time in 20 years.

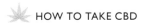

Unfortunately, research suggests that CBD does not penetrate through the dermal layer to muscles and joints below, so unless a company is using water-soluble CBD, it's unlikely the effects are more than placebo. However, applying CBD topically to calm inflammatory skin conditions appears to be a more effective use.

Advantages
Topicals give a site-specific way of using CBD for external areas of inflammation or irritation.

Disadvantages
Unrealistic expectations created by CBD companies suggest the topical application of CBD will ease pain and inflammation in joints and muscles.

Instructions for Use
Some companies recommend using generous amounts of their products and rubbing in vigorously to get around CBD's inability to penetrate the skin.

Top Tip
Always do a patch test. Just because an ingredient is 'natural' doesn't mean it can't cause irritation. Many people (including myself) find the terpene limonene irritating to their skin. So before slathering yourself in CBD body lotion, try it out on a small area of skin first.

CBD TRANSDERMAL PATCHES

CBD's poor bioavailability means research teams around the world are trying to find innovative ways to increase its absorption in the body. Transdermal patches, commonly used to deliver medications through the skin into the bloodstream, are being touted as the latest way to get more CBD bang for your buck.

However, some caution should be noted. Transdermal patches are classified as medical devices and as such are not generally used in the wellness/nutritional supplement market.

That hasn't stopped several companies in the UK from offering them to the consumer. But producing a CBD patch is more than just smothering a plaster in CBD oil. If there is to be any chance of CBD passing through the skin and entering the bloodstream, special permeability enhancers must be added.

Advantages
Patches are used in medicine because they allow a slow, gradual release of active ingredients. So, for the duration of your patch (which could last between 12 and 92 hours), there's no need to worry about whether you've remembered to take it.

Disadvantages
Information provided by CBD companies about their patches is pretty sketchy so you may well just end up with a patch smothered in CBD oil and a hole in your bank account. (Ask if it's not clear).

Instructions for Use

For best results, cleanse the skin with alcohol wipes before application. Attach the patch to a venous area, such as the inner wrist or ankle.

Top Tip

Ask the CBD company what techniques they use to make the CBD contained within the patches penetrate the skin.

CBD EDIBLES

CBD-infused hummus anyone? Or perhaps a salad with some CBD oil dressing? 2019 was the year that CBD became the star ingredient on the shelves of health-food stores like Whole Foods and Planet Organic. Adding CBD oil to our food isn't as far-fetched as it sounds, seeing as a hundred years ago we all would have had hemp, and consequently CBD, in our diet. Fast forward to the 21st century though, and selling anything 'CBD infused' can seem like little more than an excuse to double the price. That said, some CBD edibles such as CBD gummies are less faddish and can be a convenient way to incorporate CBD into your daily life.

Advantages

CBD edibles such as gummies and mints come with a fixed dosage, and are more discreet than CBD oil drops.

Disadvantages

On more gimmicky products, there's often little information about how much CBD they contain, but that doesn't stop retailers whacking up the price.

Instructions for Use

Depends on the product, but chewing for longer than you normally do with food may help absorption.

Top Tip

OK, so CBD might have great health benefits, but mixing it with sugar or artificial ingredients negates all the good work CBD might have done. So if you're going to try a CBD edible, make sure CBD features alongside other natural, wholesome ingredients.

'We should treat it in the same way as an herbal medicine – a bit harsh on the palate, but worth taking in its most natural, unadulterated form.'

CBD DRINKS

In the spirit of 'let's make a quick buck and add CBD to everything' craze, CBD has also been finding itself on the ingredients list of everything from energy drinks to alcohol and coffee. Where's the harm in that, you may ask? Personally, I have no objection to the addition of CBD to health drinks and smoothies for the more health-conscious among us. But mixing CBD with your morning coffee so you don't get the shakes or creating a CBD-infused cocktail to attract the holistic hipster crowd, contradicts the whole ethos behind CBD.

The exception lies in CBD hemp tea – adding hot water to hemp flowers – which is a relaxing alternative to herbal infusions like chamomile or valerian.

Advantages
If you're taking CBD for wellness, getting your daily CBD shot in a health drink can be a pleasant way to incorporate CBD into your life.

Disadvantages
Where do I start? CBD is often the only healthy ingredient in CBD-infused drinks. More often than not, it's not clear how much CBD they contain, so if you want accurate dosing, forget it.

Instructions for Use
Hemp flower tea: add a heaped spoonful to a cup of hot water and boil for five minutes. Open your mouth, drink, swallow and hope for the best.

Top Tip
Search out the CBD-infused health drinks, and avoid anything with caffeine, alcohol, sugar or artificial flavourings or preservatives.

Rip-off Warning: Avoid CBD Bandwagon Products
As you might have guessed by my scathing words on certain gimmicky CBD drinks and edibles, I'm not a big fan of the 'let's throw CBD in everything' approach currently finding favour.

We're talking about the likes of CBD socks, CBD pillowcases, CBD-infused mattresses and even CBD leisurewear. I kid you not. Some of these are sold as expensive novelty gifts, but others spout a load of pseudoscience in their marketing materials justifying their exorbitant prices and mere existence.

Do not be taken in.

Clothing your body in CBD-impregnated sportswear or lying on a CBD-soaked mattress at night will not make you calmer or your joints any less painful. Sorry, but it's true.

You have been warned.

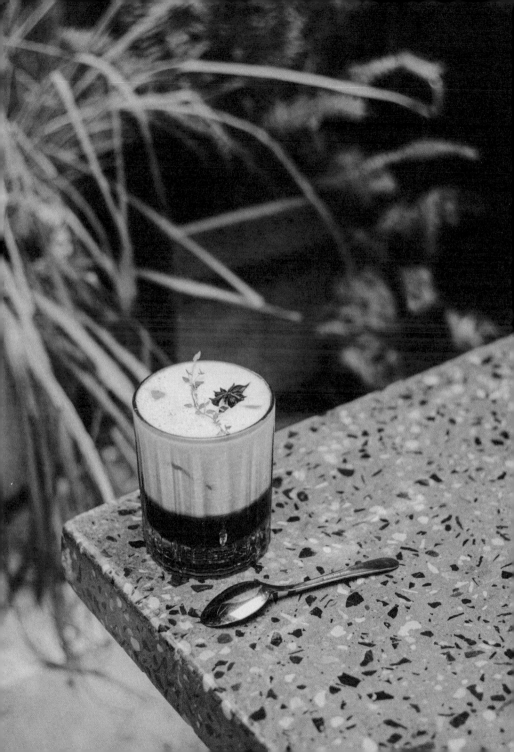

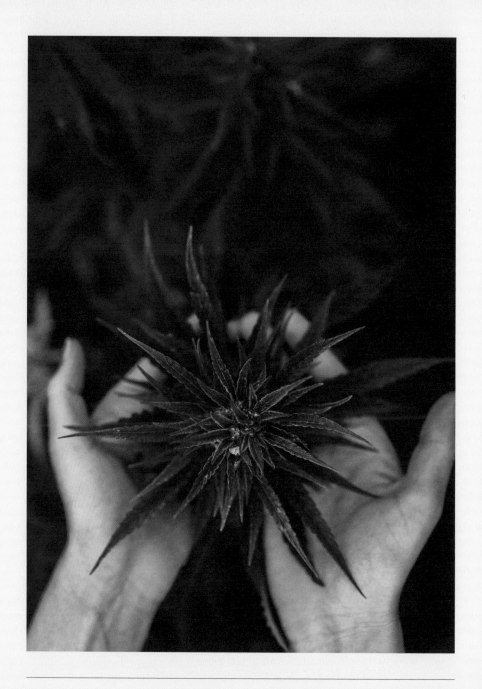

THE CBD BOOK

CHOOSING THE BEST CBD
PRODUCT FOR YOU

I used to be a cigarette smoker, but gave up after reading Alan Carr's hefty tome, *The Easy Way To Stop Smoking*. For most of the book, the reader is encouraged to continue smoking. However, by about halfway through, you're desperate to stop, if only to shut dear Alan up. I can imagine right now you may well be feeling the same, as all you really want to do is learn how to buy a decent CBD oil.

So, let's get on with it, shall we?

First things first, don't be afraid to shop for CBD oil online. Many of us struggle to trust companies selling health products online, thinking them somehow less reputable than retailers on the high street. However, with CBD, this isn't generally the case.

When CBD oil hit the scene five or so years ago, no high-street shop would touch it with a barge pole. Those early CBD companies could only be found online and because they were incredibly passionate and knowledgeable about CBD's health potential, they knew their products inside out. So, while they couldn't give medical advice, they would go the extra mile when it came to customer service.

Overall, this level of expertise and customer service continues today when you buy CBD oil online. Unfortunately, the same

cannot be said for the high street, where staff in supermarkets and chemists often know very little about the CBD products on sale. Not only that, buying from the high street is no guarantee of superior quality products. In 2020, CBD sold in a well-known pharmacy chain was found to contain no CBD at all, while products from a popular health-food store had less CBD than labelled and above the legal limit of THC.[140]

DON'T BE FOOLED BY CBD MARKETING TRICKS

That said, without the right tools and knowledge, buying CBD online can feel utterly overwhelming.

Logic would suggest that the CBD companies nearest to the top on Google must be the best. Sadly, this is not necessarily the case. I'm not knocking the CBD guys rocking the Google rankings, but most of them will have employed some nifty techniques to optimise their online content so it ranks highly on Google.

One shady technique sometimes used is setting up fake 'impartial' CBD oil review sites that miraculously link back to a company's own CBD products. Also beware of any list articles claiming to review top ten CBD oils for pain or anxiety. There is no way of saying whether one product is better than another for specific health conditions, and CBD companies have invariably paid to have their product mentioned with a backlink to their site.

A key reason CBD companies employ these tactics is to get round the regulators like the MHRA and FDA banning them from making medical claims. So while you may be yearning to find informative articles about whether CBD will cure your migraines, if a company says so on their website, you should immediately be suspicious of their credibility.

BUYING CBD – START BY FINDING A TRUSTWORTHY CBD COMPANY

Choosing which company to buy your CBD oil from is a bit like looking for a new love interest on a dating app or website. If you don't set up crucial key criteria, you will be inundated by offers of varying quality.

In CBD terms, here are a few criteria you should consider:

1. Organic
Whether for wellness purposes or to help treat symptoms of a health condition, it's important to make sure the CBD oil you take is organic certified whenever possible.

Why is this important? As well as providing us with the wonders of CBD, hemp can also remove heavy metals and radioactive toxins from polluted soil through a process called phytoremediation.[141] So imagine if the hemp used to make your CBD oil was grown on contaminated land. Thanks to hemp's soil-cleaning powers, your CBD oil would be brimming with heavy metals and goodness knows what other toxic nasties.

So, make sure you choose a company selling CBD oil made from organic certified hemp. If the products aren't organic, insist on seeing a certificate of analysis showing they are free from heavy metals, pesticides etc.

2. Transparency and Traceability
My introduction to the CBD industry came through a CBD company that controlled the whole CBD production process from seed to shelf (they grew, extracted, packaged and sold their own CBD oil). This is of tremendous benefit to the consumer, as with minimum links in the chain, it gives total traceability, greater transparency and less room for substandard products.

Because domestically grown hemp flowers cannot be used to make CBD oil in the UK, most British CBD companies source their CBD oil from mainland Europe or the United States. Perhaps they go straight to the farmers, or increasingly they might buy through a wholesale middleman.

There is nothing inherently wrong with this as long as every step is traceable. So ask yourself: how transparent is the company about where they source their CBD from? If in doubt, reach out to them and ask directly.

3. Value for Money

CBD is expensive, especially if you're taking it on an ongoing basis for a chronic illness.

That's why before you buy it's good to do a bit of homework comparing CBD oil prices. Just divide the price of comparable CBD products by the number of milligrams they contain and, hey presto, you get the price of CBD per milligram.

Make sure though you're comparing like with like. For instance, there's no point comparing the price per milligram of a water-soluble product with a standard CBD oil, as the water soluble is always going to be more expensive.

At the cheaper end of the market, some CBD companies offer CBD oils at around £0.025 per milligram, while some of the well-known American CBD products can cost as much as £0.19 per milligram; that's almost eight times the price.

However, there seems to be a well-trodden middle ground at around £0.08 per milligram, occupied by the more long-standing UK CBD companies. So if in doubt, use this as a guide price.

4. An Informative Website with No Medical Claims

You can glean a lot about a CBD company from its website. If any medical claims are made about their products, warning bells should immediately ring, even if they're referencing scientific studies to back up their claims. The MHRA has been very clear in their message that CBD cannot be said to cure or even alleviate the symptoms of any health condition.

There should also be a detailed description of each product on sale. It's not enough to say: 'Hemp oil, hemp paste (leaf and flower),' as in the case of a brand of CBD oil sold by a well-known health-food store. I would like to see not only how much CBD is in each product, but also what other cannabinoids are contained, plus, if possible, a detailed description of any terpenes.

This should all be backed up by a valid, up-to-date certificate of analysis (COA), traceable to the CBD product you are buying, and detailing not only what's in the oil, but what is not present, such as heavy metals, mould and pesticides.

5. Good Ratings on Peer Review Sites

Once upon a time you could find glowing testimonials from satisfied customers on CBD websites, waxing lyrical about the amazing health-giving benefits of their products.

Since the MHRA got involved and banned the use of testimonies on CBD websites, most companies encourage customers to write reviews on sites like Trustpilot. The good news is that CBD companies have no control over whether customers write positive or negative reviews, and once they're public, there's nothing they can do to take them down.

Comments usually cover good or bad customer service, as well as sharing personal CBD success stories. Either way, you can be fairly certain that if a company has mostly four or five stars from thousands of customers, they're doing something right.

A CBD CHECKLIST

OK, you've done your research and found a reputable CBD company. Their products are organic, competitively priced, and come with up-to-date COAs.

But which product should you actually choose?

Things to consider include:

1. Why am I Taking CBD Oil?

If you're using CBD as a nutritional supplement for overall wellness or to manage long-term symptoms of a health condition, CBD oil drops and tinctures are a good way to go as they keep a baseline level of CBD in your system.

However, if you experience breakthrough pain, sudden bouts of anxiety or panic attacks, vaping CBD can be a good add-on due to its rapid onset in the body.

2. Value for Money

Choosing a method with superior bioavailability makes sense for our pocket, as we can take less CBD to get the same result. So when possible opt for delivery methods with higher absorption rates.

3. Convenience and Practicality

That said, if you know you only get on with nutritional supplements in capsule form, buying CBD oil drops would be throwing good money after bad, even if they do have better bioavailability. So choose a CBD product that you know fits in with your lifestyle and taste.

4. Your Dosing Needs

If this is the first time you've taken CBD, it is always advisable to buy the lowest-dosage product. That way it allows you to find your optimal therapeutic dose, which is often a lot lower than you might imagine.

Let's say if you are a chronic pain sufferer, it could take as little as 10mg of CBD, three times a day, to manage your symptoms. But if you're starting on a 50mg capsule, you wouldn't have the flexibility in dosing to work that out.

Patients with more complex health needs such as neurodegenerative diseases or cancer often tend to choose higher-strength products. But ideally this should be part of a treatment plan under the supervision of a doctor experienced in prescribing cannabinoids.

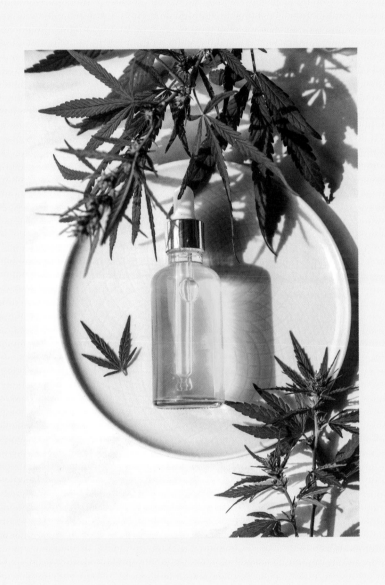

CBD DOSING – FINDING YOUR OWN SWEET SPOT

Picture the scene. After much anticipation, a little package containing your CBD oil has landed on the door mat. Once it is opened, you search for instructions telling you how much CBD to take.

Disappointingly, in the instructions for use there's some vague mention of two or three drops, three times a day, which appears to be the same advice regardless of the strength of the CBD product. So you head to the company website, which is equally unhelpful.

Hang on a sec, you think. I'm used to being told exactly how much paracetamol to take when I've got a headache, so why isn't it the same with CBD?

Here's the thing. You may be taking CBD for your headache or an arthritic hip, but it's still only classed as a nutritional supplement. Which means companies selling CBD products cannot give precise dosing suggestions, as that would constitute medical advice and would get them into trouble with the regulators.

But even if you were being prescribed CBD oil by a medical cannabis doctor, they still wouldn't be able to tell you exactly how much CBD to take because there is no standardised dose.

START LOW, GO SLOW

Doctors at the Kalapa Clinic in Barcelona, who are specialists in treating patients with cannabinoid medicine, explain:

The final effect of CBD depends on multiple factors such as weight, previous experience with cannabinoids, metabolism, pharmacological tolerance, inter-individual (genetics), differences in cannabinoid receptor function and structure, routes of administration and medical disorders. These all contribute to the difficulty in establishing a uniform schedule dosing or precise dose. Therefore, the dosage remains individualised.

The best way to find the best dosage is starting with a low dose and increasing slowly. Of course, this depends on the symptoms or underlying disease and every patient is different.

The 'start low, go slow' approach is also known as the 'up-titration method' and involves gradually building up how much CBD you take over a period of weeks. It's best to start at a sub-therapeutic level, such as 1 or 2mg, three times a day and observe the effects in the body, if any. If it's not clear from the labelling how many milligrams are in each drop of the CBD oil you have

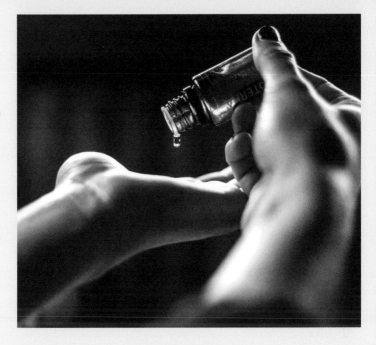

If after a week you don't feel any difference, increase the dose by a few more milligrams.

bought, simply ask the CBD company. If after a week you don't feel any difference, increase the dose by a few more milligrams. The idea is to find your own personal 'sweet spot': the point at which you feel optimal benefits from the CBD oil you are taking. To give an example, let's say you've never tried CBD before and are taking CBD to help manage stress and anxiety.

Week 1: You begin by taking 2mg, three times a day. After a week there is no change.

Week 2: You increase the dose to 4mg, three times a day. Your overall stress levels start to reduce.

Week 3: The dose is increased to 5mg, three times a day and you're feeling a lot calmer.

Week 4: You increase the dose to 6mg, three times a day and notice no further improvement.

Week 5: You reduce the dose back to 5mg, three times a day. This is your sweet spot.

While this is certainly not a dosing regime for anxiety, it does illustrate the process of finding your own dosing sweet spot. To aid this process, noting down any changes in a CBD journal (good or bad) can be helpful.

CBD DRUG INTERACTIONS

There's no getting around the fact that CBD oil is a massive disruptor to both the nutritional supplement and prescription medication market. Whether doctors like it or not, millions of patients worldwide are taking CBD for symptoms commonly treated by prescription medication. In fact, many people report being able to reduce or completely come off drugs such as antidepressants and opioids.

St John's wort is another natural remedy that has been found to be on a par with prescription antidepressant medication for mild to moderate depression. In some cases, St John's wort is even recommended by doctors, but only if patients are not taking certain kinds of medication. That's because St John's wort can interfere with drugs like oral contraceptives, making them less effective.

It's all a question of drug metabolisation. St John's wort is thought to increase the expression of the liver enzyme CYP3A4. More of this enzyme means these other medications degrade in the body more rapidly than normal, so they cannot do the job they were designed for (contraceptive pills not protecting against pregnancy, for example).

Turns out CBD may also cause some drug interactions by increasing blood plasma levels of certain medications; essentially doing the opposite to St John's wort.

CBD is broken down in the body by cytochrome P450 enzymes, in particular CYP3A4, which is responsible for metabolising 60 per cent of prescription medications.[142] However, when these medications are taken alongside CBD, the compound actually prevents other 'competing' drugs from being broken down by the CYP3A4 enzyme. Instead, higher-than-normal levels of these medications stay in the body, causing toxic build up and heightened side effects.

Depending which way you look at it, this could actually be a good thing, as this means CBD increases the bioavailability of certain drugs, potentially allowing smaller doses to be administered. However, this necessitates some kind of monitoring by doctors. In reality, few people have an open dialogue with their GP about using CBD oil, and most doctors are ill-equipped to give patients advice anyway. Plus, it's still unclear whether this interaction is dose dependent; does it only occur at the high CBD doses administered in clinical trials?

CBD AND ANTI-SEIZURE MEDICATION

The most extensive human data on CBD drug interactions comes from the various clinical trials for the purified CBD anti-epilepsy drug, Epydiolex.

Researchers found administering between 5 and 25mg of CBD per kilo of body weight daily caused higher blood plasma levels of several anti-epilepsy drugs (AEDs) including clobazam, rufinamide, topiramate, zonisamide and eslicarbazepine.[143] As a result, subjects reported increased side effects, principally sleepiness; however, these were rectified by lowering the AED dose. Worryingly, when CBD was combined with valproate, another commonly prescribed anti-seizure med, abnormal liver function was noted.[144]

Similar interactions have been found with the anticoagulant warfarin, after a patient using Epydiolex experienced elevated levels in their blood.[145] Reducing the patient's warfarin dose while still maintaining the therapeutic range for optimum blood-clotting action seemed to solve the problem. However, any changes to prescription medication should only be carried out under the guidance of a doctor.

CAN I TAKE CBD WITH MY MEDICATION?

In February 2020, the UK Food Standards Agency (FSA) announced their position on whether it's safe to take CBD alongside prescription medication. In contrast to the findings of the World Health Organisation, which deemed CBD to be generally safe and non-toxic, the FSA has advised anyone taking medication against using CBD oil.[146]

This advice was largely based on the Epidyolex studies in which paediatric epilepsy patients given high doses of purified CBD experienced more unwanted side effects caused by drug interactions. In reality, the average CBD consumer, healthy or otherwise, takes between 25 and 50mg of CBD a day, and are unlikely to suffer similar drug interactions or experience toxicity.

So, in the spirit of harm reduction, a good rule of thumb for anyone on prescription medication taking CBD is to look for 'the grapefruit warning'. Through a different mechanism, chemicals in grapefruits inhibit the CYP3A4 enzyme, leading to increased amounts of some drugs in the bloodstream. Consequently, these medications have an 'avoid grapefruit' warning on their label and include:

daliskiren (Tekturna)
alprazolam (Xanax)
amiodarone (Pacerone)
atorvastatin (Lipitor)
carbamazepine (Tegretol)
cilostazol (Pletal)
clarithromycin (Biaxin)
cyclosporine (Gengraf, Neoral)
colchicine
dronedarone (Multaq)
erythromycin (E.E.S., Eryped)
felodipine (Plendil)
fentanyl
fentanyl transdermal system
    (Duragesic Skin Patch)
fexofenadine (Allegra)
flibanserin (Addyi)
indinavir (Crixivan)
loratadine (Claritin)
losartan (Cozaar)
lovastatin

nilotinib (Tasigna)
naloxegol (Movantik)
palbociclib (Ibrance)
pazopanib (Votrient)
pimozide (Orap)
ranolazine (Ranexa)
saquinavir (Invirase, Fortovase)
sildenafil (Revatio, Viagra)
simvastatin (Zocor)
tadalafil (Adcirca, Cialis)
vardenafil (Levitra, Staxyn)
verapamil (Calan, Calan SR)
warfarin

Source www.drugs.com

Some CBD oil users take their CBD products at different times of the day to minimise potential drug interactions which manifest as dizziness, nausea, drowsiness, fatigue, diarrhoea or changes in appetite. However, if any of these symptoms do occur, stop taking your CBD oil and make an appointment to see your doctor.

The takeaway for anyone using CBD oil alongside prescription medication should be to always talk to your GP or specialist first.

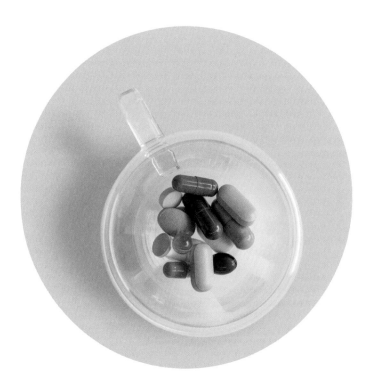

HOW TO TAKE CBD – FREQUENTLY ASKED QUESTIONS

With the CBD–drug interaction biggie out the way, let's move onto some questions commonly asked by CBD users.

1. Should I take CBD with food or on an empty stomach?
Research suggests that taking CBD alongside fatty foods increases its bioavailability.[147] While this isn't an excuse to tuck into an English breakfast every morning, it does mean taking your CBD with foods containing healthy fats such as nuts, seeds, olive oil and avocados will increase absorption.

2. How will I feel when I take CBD?
We are all different and have unique metabolisms, endocannabinoid systems and health conditions. For many of us (me included), there's no 'road to Damascus' moment the first time we take CBD. Its effects are more cumulative and one day you're like, 'Hey, I just feel super-chilled, maybe it's the CBD.' Others only notice the difference CBD is making to their lives when they stop taking it: bam! the pain, stress, anxiety levels increase again.

That said, I've heard a few cases, particularly relating to pain, where people noticed an immediate change after taking CBD. But in the end, ultimately, how each person reacts is impossible to predict.

3. Will CBD make me feel sleepy?
CBD is thought to have a biphasic effect, so as a rule, low doses cause alertness while high amounts cause somnolence. But this isn't the same for everyone.

If this is the first time you're trying CBD, it's probably a good idea to avoid taking it directly before anything important, and that includes going to bed. There's nothing worse than having insomnia, taking something you hope will help you sleep, and then feeling more wired than ever.

4. Is CBD safe during pregnancy?
So far, there hasn't been enough research into CBD's safety during pregnancy, but some evidence suggests that cannabis consumption can affect foetal development. Therefore, it is not advisable to take CBD oil during pregnancy.

5. Is it safe to give children CBD?

Most of the clinical trials for CBD have been carried out on children with drug-resistant epilepsy, so we know that CBD is well tolerated in children and infants. However, if you are considering giving your child CBD, you should discuss this with your doctor or paediatrician first.

6. Is CBD safe to take on a long-term basis?

Unfortunately, little is known about the safety of taking CBD long term. One concern is whether CBD could cause liver damage, but so far only one study on mice that were given extremely high doses of CBD suggests this might be an issue.[148] However, this study has since been widely discredited and considering the amount of CBD taken by an average consumer, there isn't anything to worry about.[149]

That said, the UK Food Standards Agency recently warned against consuming more than 70mg of CBD a day based on recent findings by the government's Committee on Toxicity.[150]

However, the Committee's conclusions were largely drawn from the Epidyolex clinical studies in which children with epilepsy were given high doses of purified CBD. This is not comparable to the significantly lower doses of whole-plant CBD oils generally taken by consumers.

7. Could CBD make me fail a drug test?

Drug tests are usually testing for THC, the psychoactive and illegal compound in cannabis. If the CBD oil you are taking complies with current regulation, you should be OK.

Unfortunately, recent reports suggest several CBD oils sold in the UK contain more than the legal limit of THC, which could theoretically mean someone could fail a drug test if they are taking these products in high doses. If you are worried about drug testing, buying a broad-spectrum CBD product should avoid any problems.

8. Is CBD Oil the same as hemp seed oil?

A common mistake made by CBD newbies is to buy hemp seed oil instead of CBD oil. Hemp seed oil is a nutritious oil with a perfect balance between essential fatty acids omega 3 and 6. Made from the seeds of the hemp plant, it does not contain CBD at all, although many CBD companies used hemp seed oil as a carrier oil to mix with hemp extract.

06

CASE STUDIES

There's a reason millions of people around the world are turning to CBD for their health. Regardless of where we are with current research, many people have experienced first hand the transformative effects of CBD oil: otherwise, the CBD market wouldn't be growing as fast as it is.

I think unless you have been in the situation of having a serious illness that cannot be satisfactorily treated by conventional medicine, it's hard to imagine how it must feel to find relief in a small bottle of rather funky-smelling oil from the cannabis plant. But this is just what has happened to innumerable patients around the world, some of whom have shared their stories with me for this book.

I am in no way suggesting that patients should forgo standard treatment in favour of CBD oil based on any of the personal accounts given here. But these cases do show how CBD oil is no mere snake oil and can in some instances return people from a point of desperation, putting them on course to reclaiming their life again.

AVA BARRY, 10

Dravet Syndrome

Ava Barry from County Cork in Ireland had her first seizure when just a baby. Her family were devastated to learn that Ava had Dravet Syndrome, a drug-resistant and very rare type of epilepsy.

Ava was put on one anti-epilepsy drug after another, until she was taking 15 tablets a day. However, none of the drugs managed to control the violent seizures Ava was having and she was experiencing a host of unpleasant side effects.

Aged just 6, Ava suffered 18 consecutive seizures in close succession, the strain of which caused a heart attack and she had to be rushed to hospital.

It was at this point that Ava's doctors effectively sent her home to die, having run out of options.

Ava's parents, Vera and Paul, had heard about Charlotte Figi, who like Ava has Dravet Syndrome but who had found significant seizure reduction from taking CBD oil.

With nothing to lose, Vera and Paul decided to try giving Ava CBD oil, choosing the same CBD oil given to Charlotte.

'I was completely terrified, of course,' says Vera. 'Even though I'd researched medical cannabis for the last four years. This is my little girl.'

Thankfully, within two months of starting CBD oil, Ava's seizures reduced by roughly 80 per cent. But the improvements in Ava's health didn't end there.

'She was standing up straighter,' recalls Vera, 'she was making more eye contact and the next thing, Ava's giggling just like the other kids at a family joke. She had never laughed like that before. She's so much better. We're seeing another side of Ava. We always knew she was beautiful and wonderful, but she's just able to put her point across a little bit more.'

Ava continues to take CBD oil alongside a small amount of THC, which she gets under prescription from the Irish government thanks to mum Vera's unrelenting campaigning. Her seizures are now completely under control and she is making excellent strides in her overall development.

EMILY WILSON, 30

Anxiety and PTSD

Emily, originally from Liverpool, lives and works in Athens, where she coordinates volunteers in a refugee camp just outside the city.

Camp life, while at times joyful, can be stressful beyond belief. Not surprising when you consider 2,800 displaced persons from countries like Syria, Afghanistan, Iraq and Iran live side by side in converted shipping containers, many still suffering from severe trauma.

After two years working on camp, Emily began to notice the strain was taking its toll.

'I remember a few times when I'd be walking,' recalls Emily, 'and I'd start to think about work and my chest would tighten and tears would roll down my cheeks. So I'd have to stop and sit by the side of the road.'

Eventually, Emily's anxiety got so crippling she felt unable to go to work.

'I couldn't get out of bed,' remembers Emily, 'because I was so scared about everything that was going on.'

So she decided to try CBD and after a few days building up the dose, Emily started to notice a positive change.

'I think the major benefit for me was it prevented the anxiety from becoming all-encompassing. It didn't take away the problems, I knew that I had to fix them, but they weren't stopping me doing things,

they were just something that were there. I also felt a deep sense of calm and my body was a lot more relaxed.

Emily also found taking CBD helped her cope with the PTSD she experienced caused by witnessing traumatic events on the refugee camp.

'I went through quite a few stages of not being able to sleep and thinking that people were camping on my terrace, and having flashbacks to certain situations that happened in the camp. The CBD oil got rid of that completely. It sent me into a very deep, carefree sleep.'

Emily is now free from anxiety, thanks to using CBD oil alongside yoga and talking therapy.

'So she decided to try CBD and after a few days building up the dose, Emily started to notice a positive change.'

JO MOSS, 44

Fibromyalgia and Chronic Fatigue Syndrome

Jo Moss has had ME and chronic fatigue since 2006. However, about six years ago she also developed fibromyalgia, becoming severely disabled and bedbound.

'Before discovering CBD,' says Jo, 'my body was in such an exhausted state that I couldn't even talk because it would set off the fight-or-flight in my body and I had really bad palpitations. I wasn't sleeping, and had horrendous pain 24/7.'

Jo first came across CBD in a fibromyalgia magazine where she saw for the first time how the condition could be linked to endocannabinoid deficiency. This was four years ago, when a handful of companies were selling CBD oil online.

'My first bottle was a low dose 2 per cent or 3 per cent CBD,' Jo recalls. 'I now know how lucky I was that the first company I came across were reputable.'

While Jo initially decided to take CBD for the unbearable pain experienced during fibromyalgia, she didn't experience any reduction for two or three months.

That's not to say she didn't notice any immediate effects.

'When your body is in fight-or-flight all the time,' Jo explains, 'you're exhausted, you're tense, which aggravates things like anxiety, but physically it was impossible to sleep. But after my first dose of CBD, it was just a calm feeling, like after a long day at work you get in the bath. And it was something quite alien because I'd been years and years in such a heightened state.'

After experimenting with higher-strength CBD oils, Jo eventually noticed her pain levels improve.

'The first time I got pain relief was quite a revelation really, it was amazing,' Jo admits.

However, Jo is quick to point out that CBD is no instant fix.

'I'm four years down the line and I've made such improvement, but it has been gradual,' she says.

'CBD gave me the chance to breathe, to relax and then rest. It took some of the pain away, the anxiety away. Over time, my body has been able to heal a lot more. Sleep is a big thing. I wasn't sleeping at all. Now I get about eight hours a night and I've been a lifelong insomniac.

'Discovering CBD was the first time my health started to improve. Before that, doctors had basically abandoned me as there was no medication they could give me. So CBD has been my only lifeline.'

NIALL MCCARTNEY, 8

Autism

Niall from Dublin was only one year old when he had a febrile convulsion, leaving him with a brain injury, severe anxiety, ongoing seizure activity, and autism. Mum Sharon noticed how, after returning from the hospital, Niall had lost all his vocabulary, and his development stagnated.

'He wasn't responding to his name, he didn't look up when the doorbell rang,' remembers Sharon. 'He had gone into his bubble. He started with repetitive behaviours and was quite violent.'

Doctors were pessimistic about Niall's future, saying that Sharon would most probably be his full-time carer for the rest of his life. With time, Niall's autism became more pronounced, and he started showing self-injurious behaviour, in particular banging his head, as well as extreme anxiety.

'We were in a chronic state in this house,' she recalls. 'All our doors and windows were locked because he was a flight risk. We could not take him anywhere because it was just too dangerous; if he got loose from my grip, he was gone. I used to refer to my house as "the prison" because I couldn't leave it.'

Niall's ongoing seizure activity meant he was at high risk of developing epilepsy, and yet there was no medication doctors could prescribe. So Sharon and her husband, who himself developed epilepsy aged 26, started researching CBD oil.

'We started giving Niall CBD oil in July 2016,' says Sharon, 'and by August, we had a different child in front of us. First of all, the self-injurious behaviour and headbanging stopped. I believe that was the seizure activity calming down. Then the hyperactivity stopped and the child could sit for five minutes. You could see his system calming down. We saw all of his senses that were in total overload come down to a normal rate.' But for Sharon, the defining moment came on day nine after starting the CBD oil when Niall had his first ever conversation, saying: 'Mammy, my head doesn't hurt and I'm not scared any more.'

Four years after starting CBD oil, Niall and his family are still seeing the benefits.

'He's the happiest, healthiest eight-year-old child, says Sharon. 'His speech has one hundred percent improved. His anxiety has totally gone.'

Despite CBD's transformative effect on Niall's health, Sharon is quick to point out that CBD is no miracle cure.

'I've been very wary of putting Niall out there as this poster boy for CBD and autism because it doesn't work for everyone. It's been a very long journey to get where we are and we've made a lot of mistakes along the way. You're not going to cure their autism. But what you're looking at is to stop "existing" within the four walls of your home and start living a life.'

THE CBD BOOK

EVE ROGINSKA, 37

Managing Steroid Withdrawal

Eve was a healthy, fit 34-year-old when she first started noticing signs that all was not well with her health. What began with tiredness, nausea and difficulty sleeping, saw Eve rushed to hospital two weeks later with near blindness, Bell's palsy and loss of balance. Doctors imagined something seriously wrong was happening to her brain, but they just couldn't find out what. So, they did what doctors tend to do when there's serious inflammation – they put her on heavy doses of intravenous steroids. Thankfully, Eve's body responded and she was eventually sent home for rehabilitation.

Still none the wiser about what was really wrong with her, Eve was kept on 55mg a day of steroids, as well as methotrexate, an immunosuppressant drug commonly given in autoimmune diseases.

However, prescribing steroids on a long-term basis should be avoided as it can lead to side effects like osteoporosis, high blood pressure, diabetes, weight gain, increased vulnerability to infection, cataracts and glaucoma, and thinning of the skin. So, gradually Eve's doctor managed to reduce her steroids dose to 20mg a day, which she remained on for about a year. Each time Eve and her doctors tried to reduce this further, she experienced debilitating withdrawal symptoms similar to coming off drugs. 'I was having terrible migraines and my painkillers

weren't working, and sometimes this lasted all day,' recalls Eve. 'I had terrible trouble sleeping. Even sleeping tablets didn't work for me any more. Then the whole day my body would feel exhausted. A lot of fatigue and a lot of muscle pain. I had brain fog continuously and kept forgetting things.'

Unable to function, Eve would have no choice but to up her steroid dose again. So Eve started doing some research, and came across CBD. She was a little concerned about how CBD would interact with the steroids and methotrexate, but her doctor advised her to stop taking the CBD if she got stomach ache or diarrhoea.

So together with her doctor, Eve began gradually reducing her steroids dose while taking 25mg of CBD oil at night. This proved to be a real game changer for minimising withdrawal symptoms.

'Three days after starting with CBD, my migraines just went away. After a week or two taking it, I felt like a normal person,' she says.

Eve has now reduced her steroids to 3mg a day and hopes to quit them completely by the summer. After a horrendous couple of years, Eve is in no doubt about the difference CBD has made to her recovery.

'I would probably have to be on steroids for the rest of my life if it wasn't for this oil. It's returned my life back.'

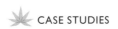

VICTORIA CLARKSON, 36

Managing Side Effects of Chemotherapy

Mum of five Victoria from West Yorkshire didn't have any dramatic warning signals of her cancer. It was a tremendous shock, then, last August when she was diagnosed with stage 4 pancreatic cancer that had spread to her lymph nodes and liver.

Not surprisingly, Victoria felt tremendously anxious when greeted with the news that she had between six months and a year to live.

Victoria had used CBD oil during a previous episode of anxiety, which she'd found helpful, so she started taking it with valerian root every night to help her sleep.

'I was getting a double whammy of two plant medicines that help with sleep and my anxiety,' she says. 'Throughout the diagnosis, if it wasn't for that, I probably wouldn't have slept. Which would obviously have made things a lot worse because if you don't sleep, your head goes.'

After her liver biopsy, Victoria began to experience more pain, so she moved onto a stronger CBD paste that also contained CBDA. The pain and discomfort only worsened when she began chemotherapy.

'I was very ill after that first chemo,' remembers Victoria. 'But I knew instantly the CBD was helping. I could feel the difference in my body.'

'When you have chemo, it feels like your insides are being burned. I could feel really sluggish and have this horrible feeling in my mouth. Within 30 minutes of taking CBD oil I felt almost human again. It's so crazy what it does.'

The benefits of taking CBD oil during chemo for Victoria have been numerous, such as aiding appetite and helping with nerve damage caused by her treatment. But for her, it's also been a way to feel empowered, during a time when your life is in other people's hands.

'CBD instantly gives you something that you can be doing for yourself. It's like handing me back my power to do everything I can to change "their" prognosis,' she says.

And it would seem that Victoria's approach, which includes CBD, a healthy diet and detoxing between rounds of chemotherapy, appears to be working.

Six months since diagnosis, and several rounds of chemo later, the cancer has gone from Victoria's lymph nodes, is barely detectable in her liver, and has shrunk from 2.5cm to 1.5cm in her pancreas. Victoria's cancer markers have also dropped from 7,000 at diagnosis to 183 in her last blood test.

Victoria's oncologist is delighted with her progress and has told her to 'keep doing whatever it is she's doing'.

JADE PROUDMAN, 40

Bowel Disease

Jade Proudman's life almost ended in 2012. After struggling with an undiagnosed form of bowel disease, the mum of three from Yorkshire collapsed and was rushed to hospital where her colon was removed in emergency surgery.

This was followed by another nine surgeries in 13 months in which she had her gallbladder and part of her liver removed, her small bowel connected to her rectum, and her abdominal cavity rebuilt with mesh after it had collapsed.

Already a fibromyalgia, ME and epilepsy sufferer, these latest surgical interventions left Jade severely disabled, housebound, in unbearable pain and suicidal.

Jade jokes how she had morphine for breakfast, codeine for lunch and tramadol for dinner, and all in all she was taking 19 different prescription medications. 'I was a toxic mess,' she admits.

Cannabis certainly wasn't on Jade's radar. But it was her husband Leslie, also her carer, who persuaded Jade to watch the CNN documentary 'Weeds', presented by Dr Sanjay Gupta.

So in 2016, Jade contacted the Stanley Brothers in Colorado who'd produced the CBD oil that so effectively reduced the seizures of Charlotte Figi, the little girl with Dravet Syndrome featured in the documentary.

'When I finally got hold of the CBD oil, I was morphine free in 48 hours. I think I cried for seven days,' remembers Jade.

No longer being on morphine made a huge difference to Jade's lucidity and overall wellbeing.

'The best way I can describe it is like somebody had cleaned my eyeballs,' she says. 'It was such a strange sensation, but it was like waking up one morning and I could see; it wasn't foggy. I could think straight.'

Thankfully, since discovering CBD, Jade has gone from needing full-time care to running her own CBD business, regularly travelling to the United States for work. She has also come off all her prescription medication and gets by on 120mg of CBD a day.

'CBD completely changed my life,' she says. 'I stopped existing and started living.'

> 'It was such a strange sensation, but it was like waking up one morning and I could see; it wasn't foggy. I could think straight.'

DAN RODWELL, 38

Crohn's Disease and Guillain-Barré Syndrome

Dan Rodwell, a businessman and father of two, had come to CBD after a friend suggested it might help manage his Crohn's disease symptoms.

'I was of the opinion that it's a snake oil, it's never going to cure me. I need clinically proven medicine for my conditions,' says Dan.

With stress triggering his Crohn's flare ups, CBD's ability to reduce Dan's anxiety meant he could get his symptoms under control, eventually coming off the medication he'd been taking for Crohn's.

However, it was Christmas 2018 when the sudden onset of a rare illness really put CBD's healing potential to the test.

One morning Dan woke up with a dead leg, which he assumed was the result of sleeping in a strange position. However, an hour later he lost sensation in his other leg, at which point he knew something more serious was happening.

Dan was rushed into hospital where he was diagnosed with Guillain-Barré Syndrome, a rare immune disorder where the immune system attacks the nervous system, thinking it's a foreign body. By that evening, Dan was in a coma lasting eight days.

'When I woke up, my body was locked,' remembers Dan, 'and I had no idea how I got to that point. The last thing I remembered was trying to roll over for a doctor to do a lumbar puncture and next I woke up with a tracheostomy and couldn't speak.'

Dosed up on fentanyl, an opioid medication 50 times stronger than heroin, Dan struggled with dark thoughts.

'Mentally I wasn't in a very good place,' he says. 'But knowing that I used CBD to treat anxiety and stress, my wife dropped some CBD sublingually, and that kind of calmed me down. You have irrational thoughts when you're in that position, so CBD basically helped me with the anxiety and the depression and gave me the strength, clear eyes and full heart to tackle the situation I was in. It also helped with the pain. I came off the painkillers pretty quickly. I thought I was going to be on them for a long time.'

Dan's recovery was expected to take between 6–18 months, but within 4 months he was back at work; something he largely attributes to taking CBD oil during his recovery.

Thankfully, Dan is now fully recovered from Guillain-Barré Syndrome and continues to take CBD oil nightly to manage his Crohn's symptoms.

LIN COXON, 71

Breast Cancer

Grandmother Lin from Derbyshire thought she'd pulled a muscle when she noticed the hard mass in her breast in May 2017. Unfortunately, a mammogram and scans confirmed it was actually stage 3 breast cancer that had spread to her lymph nodes.

Ahead of Lin lay several months of invasive treatment, including eight rounds of chemo, a mastectomy and radiotherapy, so in the eight weeks before treatment began she busied herself doing her own research.

Lin had come across Karen Roberts, another woman from Derbyshire who was cancer free after taking cannabis oil. A CBD bottle was lying around the house that had been bought for Lin's husband, so she decided to give it a go.

After ten days taking the CBD oil, Lin had an appointment with her oncologist who, after examining Lin, described the lump as 'palpable'.

'Well, you wouldn't have described the lump as palpable before,' says Lin, 'it was rock solid like the corner of a table.'

Lin carried on taking the CBD oil and every time she examined herself, the lump seemed to be shrinking.

Two days before she was due to start chemo, Lin arranged a scan privately which confirmed what she suspected: the tumour had shrunk from 33mm to 11mm. Not only

that, a further mammogram showed the tumour was no longer solid and was more like a collection of cancer cells.

This left Lin with a terrible dilemma: to go ahead with the chemotherapy or continue just taking CBD oil.

'At that point I actually cried because suddenly I was faced with a difficult decision which only I could make,' she recalls.

Lin's chemo was deferred for a week while the hospital's multidisciplinary team discussed her case. When she met with her oncologist the following week, he acknowledged what had happened to Lin was 'amazing', but said as clinicians, they still had to recommend chemotherapy.

Lin: 'So I said OK, with a stage 3 tumour left for eight weeks, what would you have expected to have seen on the scan? And he said, it wouldn't have shrunk.'

The oncologist's response was enough to convince Lin to put chemo on hold, and continue taking CBD oil instead.

'I said, if I'm prepared to take the risk, will you agree to monitor me? And he said, he would be absolutely delighted to. So, that's what they've done ever since.'

'I had a spell,' says Lin, 'when I stopped taking the oil and it grew. Not by much, by 3mm, and so I started to take the oil again

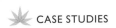

CASE STUDIES

and it shrank back. Now the size doesn't vary much at all.'

While this has been a deeply personal experience for Lin that would not necessarily be replicated in other women with breast cancer, she is clear about the impact CBD oil has had on her life.

'CBD's given me an additional three years of perfect health, to be able to carry on as normal, without having to endure chemo. I felt really well in every way. I really feel that CBD is something that does you good, especially in that period between cancer diagnosis and starting treatment.'

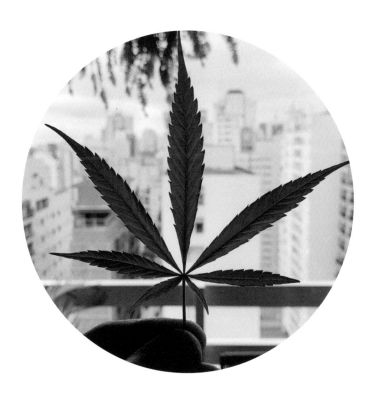

AFTERWORD

When I began writing *The CBD Book* my driving force was to create a resource that educates and informs anyone starting out on their CBD journey.

As a journalist, I'm bound to present the facts as they are and on first glance, this can appear to strengthen the argument that CBD oil is little more than a snake oil peddled by charlatans.

However, it is important to remember that for the last 70 years CBD, and cannabis in general, has been shackled by the climate of prohibition that has stymied its research.

From a personal point of view, any residual doubt I had about CBD's reported healing effects evaporated on hearing the first-hand accounts I share in the book. I did not have to cast the net very far to find these testimonies, and I am sure across the world, hundreds of thousands more ordinary people share similar experiences.

For each and every one of these cases, CBD has empowered a return to better health. This doesn't necessarily mean perfect health as we know it, but a state where some semblance of normality has returned and people are no longer reliant on prescription medication or the care of others.

And yet, the future of CBD oil remains uncertain with many fearing CBD might become a victim of its own success. Big pharma is well known for using its power

and influence to clamp down on the sale of natural alternatives to the prescription drugs it peddles. With various pharmaceutical CBD drugs in development, could their eventual approval herald a general shutting down of the CBD nutritional supplement market?

Einstein famously said 'time is an illusion', and it sure moves fast in the world of CBD. The next five years will undoubtedly see greater regulation within the CBD industry, with various systems of quality assurance already in development, which can ultimately only be of benefit to the consumer.

Time will tell whether the CBD bubble will eventually burst. For the sake of our health, I hope it doesn't.

USEFUL RESOURCES

EDUCATIONAL RESOURCES AND NEWS ABOUT CBD AND MEDICAL CANNABIS

CBD Testers www.cbdtesters.co
CBD School www.cbdschool.com
The Cannigma www.cannigma.com
Fundacion Canna
www.fundacion-canna.es/en/education
Kalapa Clinic www.kalapa-clinic.com
Leafly www.leafly.com
Project CBD www.projectcbd.org
Realm of Caring www.theroc.us

MEDICAL CANNABIS PATIENT GROUPS

Cannabis Patient Advocacy and Support
Services (CPASS) www.cannpass.org
United Patients Alliance (UPA)
www.upalliance.org

MEDICAL CANNABIS CLINICS

Kalapa Clinic www.kalapa-clinic.com
My Access Clinics
www.myaccessclinics.co.uk
The Medical Cannabis Clinics
www.themedicalcannabisclinics.com
Sapphire Medical Clinics
www.sapphireclinics.com

CBD EXPOS

The CBD Expo www.thecbdexpo.co.uk
Product Earth
www.productearthexpo.com
The CBD Show
www.rasbmedia.com/cbd-show/
The Hemp and CBD Expo
www.hempandcbdexpo.co.uk

UK CBD TRADE ASSOCIATIONS

Association for the Cannabinoid Industry
www.theaci.co.uk
British Hemp Alliance
www.britishhempalliance.co.uk
Cannabis Trades Association
www.cannabistrades.org
CannaPro www.cannapro-uk.org/
European Industrial Hemp Association
www.eiha.org

GLOSSARY

2-AG
2-Arachidonoylglycerol (2-AG) is the most abundant of the two primary endocannabinoids and binds with both CB1 and CB2 receptors.

Anandamide
Named after the Sanskrit word for bliss, anandamide was the first endocannabinoid to be discovered. It binds with both CB1 and CB2 receptors. Anandamide is produced on demand and broken down by fatty acid amide hydrolase (FAAH).

Antioxidant
Antioxidants are compounds found in many fruits and vegetables that help defend our cells from damage caused by potentially harmful molecules known as free radicals.

Apoptosis
The death of cells as a normal and controlled part of an organism's development.

Bioavailability
Bioavailability is the proportion of a substance or drug that enters the bloodstream and can be used by the body.

Broad-spectrum CBD oil
Broad-spectrum CBD oil contains CBD plus major cannabinoids and terpenes, but any THC has been removed.

Cannabidiol (CBD)
Cannabidiol is the most abundant cannabinoid in hemp. It does not create any intoxicating effect and is known to be anti-inflammatory, reduce seizures and is anxiolytic.

Cannabidiolic acid (CBDA)
CBDA is the acidic precursor of CBD and is abundantly found in the hemp plant. CBDA turns into CBD through the application of heat (a process known as decarboxylation).

Cannabinoid
A cannabinoid is a class of compound found in cannabis. There are thought to be 144 different cannabinoids, although the most abundant are THC and CBD.

Cannabis sativa
Cannabis sativa is a flowering plant indigenous to eastern Asia. Depending on the amount of THC cannabis sativa contains, it is known as marijuana or hemp. Hemp is legally defined as having less than 0.2% (0.3% in the US) THC.

CBD capsules/softgels
CBD capsules/softgels refer to CBD oil taken in capsule form, which are taken orally. These are a popular choice with people who can't tolerate the strong taste of CBD oil.

CBD edibles
CBD edibles refer to any food where CBD has been added, such as CBD gummies, CBD mints, CBD cookies, CBD cakes and CBD honey.

CBD e-liquid
CBD e-liquid is an e-liquid for e-cigarettes or vape pens usually containing PG (propylene glycol) and VG (vegetable glycerine) and infused with CBD.

CBD isolate
Crystalline pure CBD where all other cannabinoids and terpenes have been removed.

CBD oil
Hemp extract rich in CBD that has been mixed with a carrier oil, such as hemp seed oil or MCT coconut oil.

CBD suppositories
Bullet-shaped moulds filled with CBD extract mixed with coconut oil for anal or vaginal insertion.

CBD tinctures
CBD tinctures are made by steeping hemp flowers in alcohol and as such can be quite bitter to taste.

CBD topicals
CBD topicals refer to CBD products used on the skin, such as CBD creams, balms and lotions.

CBD transdermal patches
Because CBD does not penetrate through the skin, CBD transdermal patches should contain permeability enhancers in order for the CBD to reach the tissue below.

CBD vape juice
Another term for CBD e-liquid, CBD vape juice is e-liquid

containing CBD, usually in the form of CBD isolate.

CBD vape pen
A CBD vape pen is a device used to vape CBD e-liquid or concentrate and is the size and shape of a pen.

CO_2 extraction
An extraction method using high pressure CO_2 to separate cannabinoids, terpenes and flavonoids from hemp biomass.

Cortisol
Cortisol is a hormone produced in the adrenal glands. High levels may cause weight gain and high blood pressure, disrupt sleep, negatively impact mood, reduce energy levels and contribute to diabetes.

Certificate of analysis
A certificate of analysis (COA) is a document proving CBD products have undergone independent testing with specified results.

Clinical trials
Clinical trials test whether substances or medicines are safe, well tolerated and effective in humans. Gold-standard clinical trials are usually randomised double-blind placebo studies.

Cytochrome P450 enzymes
Cytochrome P450 enzymes are a group of enzymes that play a key role in the metabolism of drugs, including CBD.

Decarboxylation
Decarboxylation is the process of applying gentle heat to crude hemp extract to turn CBDA into CBD by removing a carboxyl group.

Delivery method
The route by which a medicine is delivered to the body, such as oral, sublingual, buccal, transdermal or intravenous.

Dosing sweet spot
Because there's no one-size-fits-all approach to CBD dosing, finding your sweet spot is encouraged and is the minimum amount of CBD needed to achieve a desired effect.

Endocannabinoids
Lipids made by the body that activate endocannabinoid receptors in the brain, central nervous system, immune system and organs, and which modulate biological activity.

Endocannabinoid deficiency
Suboptimal endocannabinoid levels and signalling that may

contribute to conditions typified by oversensitivity to pain, such as fibromyalgia, IBS and migraines.

Endocannabinoid system

The endocannabinoid system (ECS) comprises cannabis-like chemicals (anandamide and 2-AG) made by the body, that activate receptors (CB1 and CB2) in the brain, central nervous system, immune system and organs. Plus the enzymes that synthesise and break them down. The ECS regulates all biological activity, including appetite, sleep, reproduction, memory, mood, our immune system and cell proliferation.

Entourage effect

The proposed synergy between CBD and all the other molecules in the cannabis plant, whereby the whole is greater than the sum of its parts.

Epidyolex/Epidiolex

Purified CBD tincture approved in the United States and Europe for the treatment of drug-resistant rare types of epilepsy.

Ethanol extraction

The use of ethanol as a solvent to extract key compounds in hemp biomass.

Fatty acid amide hydrolase (FAAH)

Enzyme that metabolises anandamide in the body. CBD is known to be a FAAH inhibitor.

Flavonoids

Powerful antioxidants in almost all fruits and vegetables that are responsible for their colour.

Full-spectrum CBD oil

CBD oil retaining the full spectrum of cannabinoids, terpenes and flavonoids found in the hemp plant.

Hemp

A phenotype of Cannabis sativa containing less than 0.2 per cent THC in Europe and 0.3 per cent in the US. It has been traditionally used for its nutritious seeds and strong fibre, and as a medicine.

Hemp seed oil

Nutritious oil made from hemp seeds rich in essential fatty acids. Hemp seed oil does not usually contain CBD unless it's been used as a carrier oil in CBD products.

Homeostasis

A self-regulating process by which biological systems maintain stability while adjusting to conditions that are optimal for survival.

Lipophilic

Compounds (like CBD) that dissolve more easily in fats than water.

Marijuana

The term used to describe Cannabis sativa that contains more than the legally allowed level of THC. Has associations with recreational use, but can equally be used to describe the medical application of cannabis.

Neuroprotection

The preservation of brain cells, structures and function after strokes or in neurodegenerative diseases.

Novel foods

Foods are classified as novel if they weren't commonly consumed before 1997. When a food is added to the novel food catalogue, it must be proved safe and non-toxic before it can be sold to consumers.

Phytoremediation

A process using plants to remove, transfer, stabilise and/or destroy contaminants in the soil and groundwater.

Preclinical studies

Preclinical studies are carried out on cell cultures or animals to test a drug or procedure. They are required before clinical trials in humans can take place.

Raw hemp extract
Hemp extract that has not been decarboxylated and therefore still contains 'raw' cannabinoids such as CBDA.

Receptor
Acting like a lock on cell membranes, receptors are activated by signalling molecules such as hormones and neurotransmitters, triggering a change in the cell.

Retrospective study
Retrospective studies use past data and are observational in nature. The study outcomes have already happened at the time of its design.

Serotonin
A type of neurotransmitter produced in the brain and the gut that contributes towards feelings of wellbeing and happiness.

Serotonin 5-HT1A receptor
A serotonin-receptor subtype activated by the neurotransmitter serotonin. CBD and a number of antidepressant/anti-anxiety medications also bind with this receptor.

Terpene
A class of organic compounds found in plants and flowers responsible for their unique aromas. Certain terpenes can also cause physiological changes in the body such as relaxing the nervous system or healing wounds.

Tetrahydrocannabinol
Also known as THC, tetrahydrocannabinol is the most well-known cannabinoid in the cannabis plant due to its intoxicating effects. THC is a controlled substance and is illegal in most countries worldwide. However, it is known to have many therapeutic benefits such as being antispasmodic, antiemetic and killing cancer cells

Sativex
A cannabinoid-based drug containing roughly equal amounts of THC and CBD, approved in Europe for spasticity in multiple sclerosis.

Schedule 1 Drug
Drugs with no currently accepted medical use and a high potential for abuse. They are the most dangerous drugs of all the drug schedules, with potentially severe psychological or physical dependence.

Uptitration
The gradual increase of a drug's dose in order to reach the minimum amount to achieve optimum therapeutic results.

Vaping
The inhalation of vapour into the lungs produced by an e-cigarette or similar device. Vaping CBD allows for the best bioavailability, but comes with some safety concerns.

Water-soluble CBD
Water-soluble CBD is created by breaking CBD molecules down into nano-sized particles, making them easily dissolved in water.

Whole-plant CBD oil
A term used interchangeably with full-spectrum CBD oil to indicate a CBD oil containing the full spectrum of cannabinoids, terpenes and flavonoids found in the hemp plant.

Zero THC CBD oil
Also known as broad-spectrum CBD oil, zero THC CBD oil has had all THC removed while the other key compounds remain intact.

REFERENCES

1 Gibbs, B, Yates, D, Liebling J, O'Sullivan, S. Centre For Medical Cannabis. CBD in the UK. (June 2019).

2 Dorbian, I. CBD Market Could Pull In $16 Billion By 2025, Says Study. Forbes. (12 March 2019).

3 Gibbs, B et al (2019).

4 Brenan, M. '14% of Americans Say They Use CBD Products.' Gallup. news.gallup.com/poll/263147/americans-say-cbd-products.aspx (7 August 2019).

Part 1: The History of CBD

5 The Marihuana Tax Act of 1937.

6 United Nations Office on Drugs and Crime. Single Convention on Narcotic Drugs, 1961. www.unodc.org/unodc/en/treaties/single-convention.html.

7 The Controlled Substance Act 1970. www.dea.gov/controlled-substances-act

8 Misuse of Drugs Act 1971.

9 Pertwee, R et al. Cannabinoid pharmacology: the first 66 years. British Journal of Pharmacology, vol 147 (2006), pp. 163–171.

10 Mechoulam, R et al. 'Chronic administration of cannabidiol to healthy volunteers and epileptic patients.' Pharmacology, vol 21 (1980), pp. 175-85.

11 United States Patent Number: US 6630507. Cannabinoids as antioxidants and neuroprotectants.

12 WHO Expert Committee on Drug Dependence. CANNABIDIOL (CBD) Critical Review Report. /www.who.int/medicines/access/controlled-substances/CannabidiolCriticalReview.pdf (4–7 June 2018).

13 European Food Standards Authority. www.legislation.gov.uk/ukpga/1971/38/contents

Part 2: CBD Basics

14 Hanuš, LO et al. Phytocannabinoids: a unified critical inventory. Natural Products Reports, vol 33 (2016), pp. 1357–92.

15 Devinsky, O et al. Cannabidiol in patients with treatment-resistant epilepsy: an open-label interventional trial. The Lancet, vol 15 (2016), pp. 270–8.

16 Prud'homme, M et al. Cannabidiol as an Intervention for Addictive Behaviors: A Systematic Review of the Evidence. Substance Abuse: Research and Treatment, vol 9 (2015), pp. 33–38.

17 Linge, R et al. Cannabidiol induces rapid-acting antidepressant-like effects and enhances cortical 5-HT/glutamate neurotransmission: role of 5-HT1A receptors. Neuropharmacology, vol 103 (2016) pp. 16–26.

18 Costa, B et al. Vanilloid TRPV1 receptor mediates the antihyperalgesic effect of the nonpsychoactive cannabinoid, cannabidiol, in a rat model of acute inflammation. British Journal of Pharmacology, vol 143 (2004), pp. 247–250.

19 Ramer, R et al. COX-2 and PPAR-g Confer Cannabidiol-Induced Apoptosis of Human Lung Cancer Cells. Molecular Cancer

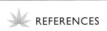

Therapeutics, vol 12 (2013), pp. 69–82.

20 Sharir, H et al. Pharmacological Characterization of GPR55, A Putative Cannabinoid Receptor. Pharmacology Therapy, vol 126 (2010), pp. 301–313.

21 Andradas, C et al. Activation of the orphan receptor GPR55 by lysophosphatidylinositol promotes metastasis in triple-negative breast cancer. Oncotarget, vol 7 (2016), pp. 47565–47575.

22 Andradas, C et al. Ibid.

23 Kaplan, B et al. The Profile of Immune Modulation by Cannabidiol (CBD) Involves Deregulation of Nuclear Factor of Activated T Cells (NFAT). Biochemical Pharmacology, vol 76 (2008), pp. 726–737.

24 Hampson, A et al. Neuroprotective antioxidants from marijuana. Annals of the New York Academy of Sciences, vol 899 (2000), pp. 274–82.

25 Russo, B. Clinical Endocannabinoid Deficiency Reconsidered: Current Research Supports the Theory in Migraine, Fibromyalgia, Irritable Bowel, and Other Treatment-Resistant Syndromes. Cannabis Cannabinoid Research, vol 1, (2016), pp. 154–165.

26 Aran, A et al. Lower circulating endocannabinoid levels in children with autism spectrum disorder. Molecular Autism vol 10, (2019).

27 Gibbs, B et al (2019).

Part 3: CBD Research

28 Ritschel et al, C. Cannabis Chemical May Treat Pancreatic Cancer, Study Finds. The Independent (21 August 2019).

29 Moreau, M et al. Flavonoid Derivative of Cannabis Demonstrates Therapeutic Potential in Preclinical Models of Metastatic Pancreatic Cancer. Frontiers in Oncology, vol 9 (2019).

30 Hurd, Y. et al. Early Phase in the Development of Cannabidiol as a Treatment for Addiction: Opioid Relapse Takes Initial Center Stage. Neurotherapeutics, vol 12 (2015), pp. 807–815.

31 Morgan, C. et al. Cannabidiol reduces cigarette consumption in tobacco smokers: preliminary findings. Addictive Behaviors, vol 38 (2013), pp. 2433–6.

32 Morgan, C. et al. Cannabidiol Attenuates the Appetitive Effects of Tetrahydrocannabinol in Humans Smoking Their Chosen Cannabis. Neuropsychopharmacology, vol 35 (2010), pp. 1879–1885.

33 Crippa, J. et al. Cannabidiol for the treatment of cannabis withdrawal syndrome: a case report. Journal of Clinical Pharmacy and Therapeutics, vol 38 (2013), pp. 162–4.

34 UK Research and Innovation. Cannabidiol: a novel treatment for cannabis dependence? University College London.

35 Linge, R et al (2016).

36 Hillard, C et al. Stress Regulates Endocannabinoid-CB1 Receptor Signaling. Seminars in Immunology, vol 26 (2014) pp. 380–388.

37 Bergamaschi M et al, Cannabidiol Reduces the Anxiety Induced by Simulated Public Speaking in Treatment-Naïve Social Phobia Patients. Neuropsychopharmacology, vol 36 (2011), pp. 1219–1226

38 Masataka, N et al. Anxiolytic Effects of Repeated Cannabidiol Treatment in Teenagers With Social Anxiety Disorders. Frontiers in Psychology, (2019).

39 Shannon, S et al. Cannabidiol in Anxiety and

Sleep: A Large Case Series. The Permanente Journal, vol 23 (2019), pp. 18-41.

40 Aran, A et al (2019).

41 Bar-Lev Schleider, L. et al. Real life Experience of Medical Cannabis Treatment in Autism: Analysis of Safety and Efficacy. Scientific Reports, vol 9 (2019) pp. 200.

42 Aran, A. et al. Brief Report: Cannabidiol-Rich Cannabis in Children with Autism Spectrum Disorder and Severe Behavioral Problems-A Retrospective Feasibility Study. Journal of Autism and Developmental Disorders, vol 49 (2019), pp. 1284-1288.

43 ClinicalTrials.gov. Cannabinoids for Behavioral Problems in Children With ASD (CBA).

44 Kaplan, B. et al. The Profile of Immune Modulation by Cannabidiol (CBD) Involves Deregulation of Nuclear Factor of Activated T Cells (NFAT). Biochemical Pharmacology, vol 76 (2008), pp. 726–737.

45 Vuolo, F. et al. Evaluation of Serum Cytokines Levels and the Role of Cannabidiol Treatment in Animal Model of Asthma. Mediators of Inflammation, (2015), pp. 538670.

46 Kumagai, S. et al. Pathological roles of oxidative stress in autoimmune diseases. The Japanese Journal of Clinical Pathology, vol 51(2003), pp. 126–32.

47 Elliot, D. et al. Cannabidiol Attenuates Experimental Autoimmune Encephalomyelitis Model of Multiple Sclerosis Through Induction of Myeloid-Derived Suppressor Cells. Frontiers in Immunology, vol 9 (2018), pp. 1782.

48 Lehmann, C. et al. Experimental cannabidiol treatment reduces early pancreatic inflammation in type 1 diabetes. Clinical Hemorheology and Microcirculation, vol 64 (2016), pp. 655–662.

49 Lee, W. et al. Cannabidiol Limits T Cell-Mediated Chronic Autoimmune Myocarditis: Implications to Autoimmune Disorders and Organ Transplantation. Molecular Medicine, vol 22 (2016), pp. 136-146.

50 ClinicalTrials.gov. A Phase 2a Study to Evaluate the Safety and Efficacy of Cannabidiol Only as Maintenance Therapy and Steroid Sparing in Patients With Stable Autoimmune Hepatitis.

51 ClinicalTrials.gov. A Phase 2a Study to Evaluate the Safety, Tolerability and Efficacy of Cannabidiol as a Steroid-sparing Therapy in Steroid-dependent Crohn's Disease Patients.

52 Hasenoehrl, C. et al. GPR55-Mediated Effects in Colon Cancer Cell Lines. Medical Cannabis and Cannabinoids vol 2 (2019), pp. 22–28.

53 Ramer, R. et al. COX-2 and PPAR-γ confer cannabidiol-induced apoptosis of human lung cancer cells. Molecular Cancer Therapeutics, vol 12 (2013), pp. 69-82.

54 Shrivastava, A. et al. Cannabidiol induces programmed cell death in breast cancer cells by coordinating the cross-talk between apoptosis and autophagy. Molecular Cancer Therapeutics, vol 10 (2011), pp. 1161–72.

55 Gallily, R. et al. Gamma-irradiation enhances apoptosis induced by cannabidiol, a non-psychotropic cannabinoid, in cultured HL-60 myeloblastic leukemia cells. Leukemia and Lymphoma, vol 44 (2003), pp. 176–73.

56 Fisher, T. et al. In vitro and in vivo efficacy of non-psychoactive cannabidiol in neuroblastoma. Current Oncology, vol 23 (2016), pp. 15–22.

57 Ligresti, A. et al. Anti-tumor activity of plant cannabinoids with emphasis on the effect of cannabidiol on human breast carcinoma. Journal of Pharmacology and Experimental

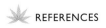

Therapeutics, vol 318 (2006), pp. 1375–87.

58 McAllister, S. et al. Cannabidiol as a novel inhibitor of Id-1 gene expression in aggressive breast cancer cells. Molecular Cancer Therapeutics, vol 6 (2007), pp. 2921–7.

59 Solinas, M. et al. Cannabidiol inhibits angiogenesis by multiple mechanisms. British Journal of Pharmacology, vol 167 (2012), pp. 1218–1231.

60 Kenyon, J. Report of Objective Clinical Responses of Cancer Patients to Pharmaceutical-grade Synthetic Cannabidiol. Anticancer Research, vol 38 (2018).

61 Liu, W. et al. Anticancer effects of phyto-cannabinoids used with chemotherapy in leukaemia cells can be improved by altering the sequence of their administration. International Journal of Oncology, vol 51 (2017), pp. 369–377.

62 ClinicalTrials.gov. TN-TC11G (THC+CBD) Combination With Temozolomide and Radiotherapy in Patients With Newly-diagnosed Glioblastoma.

63 Project CBD. Cultivating Wellness Survey www.projectcbd.org/reports/cultivating-wellness/summary (2019).

64 Sagy, I et al. Safety and Efficacy of Medical Cannabis in Fibromyalgia. Journal of Clinical Medicine, vol 8(2019), pp. 807.

65 National Institute for Health and Care Excellence. www.nice.org.uk/guidance/ng144/chapter/Recommendations#chronic-pain (November 2019).

66 Malfait, A. et al. The nonpsychoactive cannabis constituent cannabidiol is an oral anti-arthritic therapeutic in murine collagen-induced arthritis. Proc Natl Acad Sci, vol 97 (2000), pp. 9561–6.

67 Philpott, H. et al. Attenuation of early phase inflammation by cannabidiol prevents pain and nerve damage in rat osteoarthritis. Pain, vol 158 (2017) pp. 2442–2451.

68 Hammell, D. et al. Transdermal cannabiiol reduces inflammation and pain-related behaviours in a rat model of arthritis. European Journal of Pain, vol 20 (2016) pp. 936–948.

69 Xu, D. et al. The Effectiveness of Topical Cannabidiol Oil in Symptomatic Relief of Peripheral Neuropathy of the Lower Extremities. Current Pharmaceutical Biotechnology, (2019).

70 Kaplan, B. et al. The Profile of Immune Modulation by Cannabidiol (CBD) Involves Deregulation of Nuclear Factor of Activated T Cells (NFAT). Biochemical Pharmacology 76. (2008) pp. 726–737.

71 Nuki, P. Can I take ibuprofen to treat coronavirus symptoms? Expert advice on which painkillers you should take – and which to avoid. The Telegraph. 29 March 2020.

72 Shi Y et al. COVID-19 infection: the perspectives on immune responses. Cell Death and Differentiation (2020).

73 Hill, M et al. Serum Endocannabinoid Content is Altered in Females with Depressive Disorders: A Preliminary Report. Pharmacopsychiatry vol 41, (2008), pp. 48–53.

74 Dincheva, I. et al. FAAH genetic variation enhances fronto-amygdala function in mouse and human. Nature Communications vol 6, (2015), pp. 6395.

75 David A. Raichlen et al, Wired to run: exercise-induced endocannabinoid signaling in humans and cursorial mammals with implications for the 'runner's high'. Journal

of Experimental Biology, vol 215 (2012) pp. 1331–1336.

76 Shoval, G. et al, Prohedonic Effect of Cannabidiol in a Rat Model of Depression. Neuropsychobiology, vol 73 (2016), pp. 123–9.

77 Pamplona, F et al. Potential Clinical Benefits of CBD-Rich Cannabis Extracts Over Purified CBD in Treatment-Resistant Epilepsy: Observational Data Meta-analysis. Frontiers in Neurology, (2018).

78 Geffery, A et al. Drug-drug interaction between clobazam and cannabidiol in children with refractory epilepsy. Epilepsia, vol 56 (2015), pp. 1246–51

79 Stanley, C. et al. Is the cardiovascular system a therapeutic target for cannabidiol? British Journal of Clinical Pharmacology, vol 75 (2013), pp. 313–22.

80 Walsh, S. et al. Acute administration of cannabidiol in vivo suppresses ischaemia-induced cardiac arrhythmias and reduces infarct size when given at reperfusion. British Journal of Pharmacology, vol 160 (2010), pp.1234–42.

81 O'Sullivan, S. et al. A single dose of cannabidiol reduces blood pressure in healthy volunteers in a randomized crossover study. JCI Insight, vol 2 (2017).

82 Sultan, SR, O'Sullivan, SE, England, TJ. The effects of acute and sustained cannabidiol dosing for seven days on the haemodynamics in healthy men: A randomised controlled trial. Br J Clin Pharmacol. 2020; 1–14. www.doi.org/10.1111/bcp.14225.

83 ClinicalTrials.gov. Cannabidiol in Patients With Heart Failure Failure in AHA/ACC Stages A-C. CBD For Wellness.

84 Hasenoehrl, C. et al. Cannabinoids for treating inflammatory bowel diseases: where are we and where do we go? Expert Review of Gastroenterology and Hepatology, vol 11 (2017), pp. 329–337.

85 Pagano, E. et al. An Orally Active Cannabis Extract with High Content in Cannabidiol attenuates Chemically-induced Intestinal Inflammation and Hypermotility in the Mouse. Frontiers in Pharmacology, vol 4 (2016), pp. 341.

86 Naftali, T. et al. Cannabis induces clinical response but no endoscopic response in Crohn's disease patients. United European Gastroenterology Journal, vol 6 (2018).

87 ClinicalTrials.gov. A Pilot Study of GWP42003 in the Symptomatic Treatment of Ulcerative Colitis (GWID10160).

88 ClinicalTrials.gov. A Phase 2a Study to Evaluate the Safety, Tolerability and Efficacy of Cannabidiol as a Steroid-sparing Therapy in Steroid-dependent Crohn's Disease Patients.

89 United States Patent Number: US 6630507. Cannabinoids as antioxidants and neuroprotectants.

90 Aymerich, M. et al. Cannabinoid pharmacology/therapeutics in chronic degenerative disorders affecting the central nervous system. Biochemical Pharmacology, vol 157 (2018), pp. 157: 67–84.

91 Esposito, G. et al. Cannabidiol in vivo blunts β-amyloid induced neuroinflammation by suppressing IL-1β and iNOS expression. British Journal of Pharmacology, vol 151 (2007), pp. 1272–1279.

92 ClinicalTrials.gov. Cannabidiol Solution for the Treatment of Behavioral Symptoms in Older Adults With Alzheimer's Dementia (CBD).

93 Zuardi, A. et al. Cannabidiol for the treatment

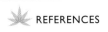

of psychosis in Parkinson's disease. Journal of Psychopharmacology, vol 23 (2009), pp. 979–83.

94 Chaggas, M. et al. Cannabidiol can improve complex sleep-related behaviours associated with rapid eye movement sleep behaviour disorder in Parkinson's disease patients: a case series. Journal of Clinical Pharmacy and Therapeutics, vol 39 (2014), pp. 564–6.

95 "Parkinson's patients to receive cannabidiol treatment in pioneering clinical trial." www.parkinsons.org.uk/news/parkinsons-patients-receive-cannabidiol-treatment-pioneering-clinical-trial-0 (14 October 2019).

96 ClinicalTrials.gov. A Study of Tolerability and Efficacy of Cannabidiol on Motor Symptoms in Parkinson's Disease.

97 Martins de Faria, S. et al. Effects of acute cannabidiol administration on anxiety and tremors induced by a Simulated Public Speaking Test in patients with Parkinson's disease. Journal of Psychopharmacology, vol 34 (2020), pp.189–196.

98 Elliot, D. et al. Cannabidiol Attenuates Experimental Autoimmune Encephalomyelitis Model of Multiple Sclerosis Through Induction of Myeloid-Derived Suppressor Cells. Frontiers in Immunology, vol 9 (2018); pp. 1782.

99 Giuffrida, A. et al. Cerebrospinal anandamide levels are elevated in acute schizophrenia and are inversely correlated with psychotic symptoms. Neuropsychopharmacology, vol 29 (2004) pp. 2108-14.

100 Schubart, C. et al. Cannabis with high cannabidiol content is associated with fewer psychotic experiences. Schizophrenia Research, vol 130 (2011), pp. 216–21.

101 Leweke, F. et al. Cannabidiol enhances anandamide signaling and alleviates psychotic symptoms of schizophrenia. Translational Psychiatry, vol 2 (2012) pp. 94.

102 McGuire, P. et al. Cannabidiol (CBD) as an Adjunctive Therapy in Schizophrenia: A Multicenter Randomized Controlled Trial. American Journal of Psychiatry, vol 175 (2018), pp. 225–231.

103 Boggs, D. et al. The effects of cannabidiol (CBD) on cognition and symptoms in outpatients with chronic schizophrenia a randomized placebo controlled trial. Psychopharmacology, vol 235 (2018), pp. 1923–1932.

104 Di Marzo, V. et al. Endocannabinoids: endogenous cannabinoid receptor ligands with neuromodulatory action. Trends in Neuroscience vol 21 (1998), pp. 521–8.

105 Hill, M et al. Reductions in circulating endocannabinoid levels in individuals with post-traumatic stress disorder following exposure to the World Trade Center attacks. Psychoneuroendocrinology, vol 38 (2013), pp. 2952–61.

106 Neumeister, A. The endocannabinoid system provides an avenue for evidence-based treatment development for PTSD. Depression and Anxiety, vol 30 (2013), pp. 93–6.

107 Elms, L. et al. Cannabidiol in the Treatment of Post-Traumatic Stress Disorder: A Case Series. Journal of Alternative and Complementary Medicine, vol 24 (2019), pp. 392–397.

108 Raymundi, A. et al. A time-dependent contribution of hippocampal CB1, CB2 and PPARγ receptors to cannabidiol-induced disruption of fear memory consolidation. British Journal of Pharmacology, vol 177 (2020), pp. 945–957.

109 Oláh, A. et al. Cannabidiol exerts sebostatic and anti-inflammatory effects on human

sebocytes. Journal of Clinical Investigation, vol 124 (2014), pp. 3713–24.

110 Van Klingeren, B. et al. Antibacterial activity of delta9-tetrahydrocrocannabinol and cannabidiol. Antonie Van Leeuwenhoek, vol 42 (1976), pp. 9–12.

111 Palmieri, B. et al. A therapeutic effect of cbd-enriched ointment in inflammatory skin diseases and cutaneous scars. Clinica Terapeutica, vol 170 (2019), pp. 93–99.

112 Hayakawa, K. et al. Therapeutic Potential of Non-Psychotropic Cannabidiol in Ischemic Stroke. Pharmaceuticals, vol 3 (2010), pp. 2197–2212.

113 Ceprián, M. et al. Cannabidiol reduces brain damage and improves functional recovery in a neonatal rat model of arterial ischemic stroke. Neuropharmacology, vol 116 (2017), pp. 151–159.

114 ClinicalTrials.gov. Hemp-Derived Botanical Dietary Supplementation During Recovery From Brain Injury.

115 The Washington Post. Do no harm: Retired NFL players endure a lifetime of hurt.

116 Biles, M. CBD for Brain-Damaged Babies. Project CBD (June 2019).

117 Martinez-Orgado, J. et al. Neuroprotective Effects of Cannabidiol in Hypoxic Ischemic Insult. The Therapeutic Window in Newborn Mice. CNS and Neurological Disorders Drug Targets, vol 16 (2017), pp. 102–108.

Part 4: CBD for Wellness

118 Sharir, H et al. Pharmacological Characterization of GPR55, A Putative Cannabinoid Receptor. Pharmacology Therapy, vol 126 (2010), pp. 301–313.

119 Mental Health Foundation. "Stressed nation: 74% of UK 'overwhelmed or unable to cope' at some point in the past year." www.mentalhealth.org.uk/news/stressed-nation-74-uk-overwhelmed-or-unable-to-cope-some-point-past-year (May 2018).

120 The American Institute of Stress. "42 Worrying Workplace Stress Statistics." www.stress.org/42-worrying-workplace-stress-statistics (25 September 2019).

121 Morena, M. et al. Neurobiological Interactions Between Stress and the Endocannabinoid System. Neuropsychopharmacology, vol 41 (2016) pp. 80–102.

122 Tawakol, A. et al. Relation between resting amygdalar activity and cardiovascular events: a longitudinal and cohort study. The Lancet, vol 389 (2017), pp. 834–845.

123 O'Sullivan, S. et al (2017).

124 Colten, H et al. Sleep Disorders and Sleep Deprivation: An Unmet Public Health Problem. National Academies Press (US (2006).

125 Spiegel, K. et al. Impact of sleep debt on metabolic and endocrine function. The Lancet, vol 354 (1999), pp. 1435-9.

126 Moreau, M et al (2019).

127 Zuardi, A. et al. Effect of cannabidiol on plasma prolactin, growth hormone and cortisol in human volunteers. Brazilian Journal of Medical and Biological Research, vol 26 (1993) pp. 213-7.

128 Project CBD. Cultivating Wellness Survey. Available at: www.projectcbd.org/reports/cultivating-wellness/summary (2019).

129 The Brightfield Group, 'Understanding Cannabidiol'.

130 'Usage of dietary supplements among U.S. adults in 2018, by gender.' Available at: www.statista.com/statistics/308333/

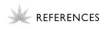

dietary-supplement-usage-us-adults-by-gender/.

131 Project CBD. Cultivating Wellness Survey. Available at: www.projectcbd.org/reports/ cultivating-wellness/summary (2019).

132 Prohibition Partners. Disrupting Beauty Report. www.prohibitionpartners.com/ reports/#disrupting-beauty (January 2020).

Part 5: How To Take CBD

133 Ben-Shabat, S. et al. An entourage effect: inactive endogenous fatty acid glycerol esters enhance 2-arachidonoyl-glycerol cannabinoid activity. European Journal of Pharmacology, vol 353 (1998), pp. 23–31.

134 Russo, E. Taming THC: potential cannabis synergy and phytocannabinoid-terpenoid entourage effects. British Journal of Pharmacology, vol 163 (2011), pp. 1344–1364.

135 Hampson, A et al (2000).

136 Blasco-Benito, S. et al. Appraising the 'entourage effect': Anti-tumor action of a pure cannabinoid versus a botanical drug preparation in preclinical models of breast cancer. Biochemical Pharmacology, vol 157 (2018) pp. 285–293.

137 Gibbs, B et al (2019).

138 Cannabinoid Testing In Europe – List of testing Laboratories www.cbdoileurope.com/ cbd-testing/cannabinoid-testing-in-europe-list-of-testing-laboratories/.

139 Williams, M. et al. Effects of Model, Method of Collection, and Topography on Chemical Elements and Metals in the Aerosol of Tank-Style Electronic Cigarettes. Scientific Reports, vol 9 (2019), Article number: 13969.

140 What's really in cannabis-based health products? BBC TV.

141 Ahmad, R. et al. Phytoremediation Potential of Hemp (Cannabis sativa L.): Identification and Characterization of Heavy Metals Responsive Genes. Clean Soil Air Water, Vol 44 (2016) pp. 195–201.

142 Adrian Devitt-Lee. CBD-Drug Interactions: The Role of Cytochrome P450. Project CBD, (2015).

143 Iffland, K. et al. An Update on Safety and Side Effects of Cannabidiol: A Review of Clinical Data and Relevant Animal Studies. Cannabis and Cannabinoid Research, vol 2 (2017), pp. 139–154.

144 Chang, B. Cannabidiol and Serum Antiepileptic Drug Levels: The ABCs of CBD With AEDs. Epilepsy Currents, vol 18 (2018) pp. 33–34.

145 Grayson, L. et al. An interaction between warfarin and cannabidiol, a case report. Epilepsy and Behaviour Case Reports, vol 9 (2018), pp. 10–11.

146 'Food Standards Agency sets deadline for the CBD industry and provides safety advice to consumers.' (13 February 2020).

147 Birnbaum, A. et al. Food effect on pharmacokinetics of cannabidiol oral capsules in adult patients with refractory epilepsy. Epilepsia, vol 60 (2019).

148 Ewing, L. et al. Hepatotoxicity of a Cannabidiol-Rich Cannabis Extract in the Mouse Model. Molecules Vol 24 (2019), pp. 1694.

149 Ewing, L. et al. Hepatotoxicity of a Cannabidiol-Rich Cannabis Extract in the Mouse Model. Molecules Vol 24 (2019), pp. 1694.

150 Adrian Devitt-Lee. "Is CBD Toxic to the Liver." Project CBD. www.projectcbd.org/ science/cbd-toxic-liver (11 July 2019).

ACKNOWLEDGEMENTS

From the Author

My journey towards writing this book started with a conversation in my kitchen in Seville with my friend Ana, who shared how the cannabis oil her mum had received in the last few months of her life had not only controlled her pain, but had allowed her to die with dignity. There and then I promised to her and the universe, that I would use my writing to shine a light on the healing powers of the cannabis plant. So my first heart-felt thanks must go to Ana and her mum Jose.

Turned out the universe was indeed listening, as just two weeks later I was offered a job as a writer for the CBD company Endoca after meeting them at a hemp fair. I will be forever grateful to Ian David Chapman for the encouragement and mentoring I received from him while at Endoca and to Demi Pradolin, my digital marketing partner in crime, who out-geeks even me when it comes to CBD and cannabis.

Back then, my point of reference for educating myself in all things cannabis was Project CBD, the not-for-profit educational resource based in California and co-founded by Martin A. Lee. Becoming a regular Project CBD contributing writer has been one of my 'cannabis career' highlights and I owe a special thanks to Martin for giving *The CBD Book* the 'once over' and for his continued support, and to Helen Rochester from HarperCollins for seeing the potential in me as an author and for her trust and enthusiasm throughout the process of writing this book.

My total appreciation, and respect must go to all the patients and carers who have generously shared their stories with me in this book and over the years. I am in total awe of your courage, strength and tenacity. I am also hugely grateful to a select bunch of scientists and doctors, in particular Professors Manuel Guzmán and Jose Javier Fernandez Ruiz from the Complutense University in Madrid, Dr Wai Liu at St Georges in London, and Dr Mariano Garcia de Palau from the Kalapa Clinic, who have patiently answered every question I've posed to them in my research over the years.

Thanks too goes to my family and friends, especially Nichola Schwarz who truly knows how to show up when it matters, and my partner Miguel, for still getting excited for me when I'd forgotten how amazing this project was.

And finally, to my mum. You weren't exactly convinced when your daughter found her calling in cannabis. But I know you approve now, even if you're not here to tell me in person.

IMAGE CREDITS

Images © Shutterstock.com: 6 Apple_Martini; 15 Karolis Kavolelis; 25 Infinity Time; 28 HQuality; 37 MexChriss; 105 IRA_EVVA.

Images courtesy of Unsplash: 8 Matthew Brodeur; 19 Brett Jordan; 20 Kimzy Nanney; 31 Motoki Tonn; 39 Matthew Henry; 44 Nathan-Dumlao Xi; 49 Amplitude Magazin; 53 Freestocks; 58 Element5 Digital; 61 Jannes Jacobs; 65, 92 Enecta Cannabis Extracts; 67 Hailey Reed; 69 Gemma Chua-Tran; 76 Michelle; 79 Katarzyna Grabowska; 80 Alex Loup; 82 Pharma Hemp Complex; 87 Michal Wozniak; 100 Hoan Vo; 102 Davide Ragusa; 109 Christin Hume; 112 Adam Niescioruk; 126 Linoleum Magazine; 142 Robert Nelson.

INDEX

HarperCollinsPublishers
1 London Bridge Street
London SE1 9GF
www.harpercollins.co.uk

First published by Thorsons, an imprint of HarperCollinsPublishers 2020.

1 3 5 7 9 10 8 6 4 2

Copyright © Mary Biles 2020.

Mary Biles asserts her moral right to be identified as the author of this work.

A catalogue record of this book is available from the British Library.

ISBN: 978-0-00-840306-5

Cover and interior design by Studio Polka..

Printed and bound in Latvia by PNB Print Ltd..

This book is produced from independently certified FSC™ paper to ensure responsible forest management.

For more information visit: www.harpercollins.co.uk/green